The Transform Diet

Transforming the world one body at a time starting with you

Brett Salisbury

iUniverse, Inc.
New York   Bloomington

The Transform Diet
Transforming the world one body at a time starting with you

iUniverse books may be ordered through booksellers or by contacting:

iUniverse
1663 Liberty Drive
Bloomington, IN 47403
www.iuniverse.com
1-800-Authors (1-800-288-4677)

ISBN: 978-0-595-51569-1 (pbk)
ISBN: 978-0-595-50497-8 (cloth)
ISBN: 978-0-595-61947-4 (ebk)

Printed in the United States of America

Cover photo by Chip Morton Photography in Temecula, California.

iUniverse Rev. 12/2/08

Contents

To my mother and father

My father died on July 11, 2007, after being diagnosed nine months earlier with mesothelioma cancer—a cancer caused by exposure to asbestos. His death came as a shock to all of us; he had been a healthy sixty-seven-year-old man. Just months earlier, he had competed in the Senior Olympics and won four gold medals. An avid weight lifter who rarely ate properly, he always led by example and hardly ever missed a workout, even up to his death. He was the epitome of what a human being should be.

Unfortunately, it took this tragic event for me to reevaluate my life and give me the strength to write this book. Knowing my calling on this earth has always been the messenger, I'm grateful now that you will know what I have learned about diet and exercise.

My mother is now sixty-nine years old. She is an avid reader who has the biggest heart there is. She has always been honest with people and has allowed me to be who I wanted to be. My mom is one tough lady. She has been a rock since the death of my father and has learned to survive without him. I'm forever grateful for her, and love her more than words can say.

Acknowledgments

I want to thank Isa and my son Elvis. I'm grateful for them and would not be where I am today without their support.

I'm also thankful for my sister Darla and brother Curt for their support and feedback no matter what decisions I have made, good or bad.

To my childhood friend, Glen Dupras who has always stood by my side.

To Donald Trump and Bill Zanker for writing *Thinking Big and Kicking Ass*. It was literally days after reading their book that I decided to act on everything I had ever known.

To Rhonda Byrne for writing *The Secret*; it confirmed my belief that we can have anything in life that we want.

To Eckhart Tolle for writing *The Power of Now*, teaching me how to truly let go of the past for it has little use, ignore the future and live in this very moment. By living in the now is where true peace and happiness are felt.

My deepest thanks to Charlie and Marv Heintschel. My friends and business partners who have listened to my vision and felt my passion to help make this lifelong dream finally come true.

Introduction

How many books are we going to continue to read that tell us how much folic acid and Vitamin C we need? It seems every diet book on the shelf is filled with information on how foods affect our internal body, with very few breaking down the external effects. That being said, for the past twenty plus years, I have waited for someone to come along and write a book that tells us to the gram, ounce and minute how much protein, carbohydrates, fat, water intake, meals and type of workout we need each day to have an entire transformation, answering those questions specifically. I wanted to focus on the latest research from the best institutions in the world in an unbiased manner, weeding fact from fiction. I stayed away from special interest groups or doctors who have ulterior motives.

To my amazement, twenty-three years later, that book has still not been written the way it should be. I start with this promise: this will be the most detailed, structured, precise and easy-to-understand diet book that you have ever read.

What qualifies me to write this book?

I have lived on two continents and traveled the world as a working model and professional football player. I have transformed some of the greatest male and female bodies on this planet.

At age sixteen, I knew I had a knack for writing diet plans. I was giving instructions to my brother's roommates who played on the 1985 USC football team. They were glued to their seats as I described what foods were best for burning body fat while maintaining lean muscle. I knew right then and there that it was my calling in life.

After high school, I had the privilege of studying at two of the finest institutions in the nation. In 1986, I received a full scholarship to Brigham Young University; four years later, a full-ride to the University of Oregon. Two years later, I finished third for the Harlon Hill Award at Wayne State College in Nebraska—Division II's version of the Heisman Trophy. I was a unanimous

All-American pick as a quarterback and earned the Nebraska offensive Player of the Year award.

After college, I played football professionally in Europe and received Player of the Year honors for three consecutive seasons. I went on to work as a successful model in Scandinavia and Milan, learning every diet trick of the trade. I have worked with the two highest-paid male models in the world: Marcus Schenkenberg and Michael Bergin. In 2002, I was fortunate to earn the title "Male Supermodel" from ModelMax senior editor Jed Medina.

I am a certified sports nutritionist with more than twenty-three years of expertise. I have studied nutrition and exercise physiology with some of the greatest minds and thinkers on earth. I'm grateful for the opportunity to share this knowledge with you.

Quite frankly, as proud as I am to have been born in this country, I'm tired of hearing how obese we are in America. We have more cutting-edge technology than we know what to do with. The rest of the world looks to us as the leader. Yet sadly, we are the fattest nation on the planet.

The good news is that Americans hate to lose. When it comes to dieting and exercise, we have more people trying to find the truth. With so much advice out there, it's tough to weed out what is right and wrong. That is why I wrote this book.

In April 2008, I was working in an office behind a desk knowing that my calling in life was to write this book. I'm on a mission to help transform the world—starting with the United States. After the bottle tree picture was taken on the back of this book, I went home with my family and laughed at the digital pictures of how heavy I looked. As we studied each picture, I was shocked at what my waistline had become. At six-foot-two and nearly 260 pounds, I had uncontrollable belly fat, but also the full knowledge of how to change my body. Later that night, as we were getting ready to watch TV, my ex-wife made a comment that I will never forget. She said, "Hey fatty, can you hand me the remote?"

The comment blew me away and put me back on track to writing this much-needed book. I made it very clear it would be the last time she would ever say that to me. I explained to her that I was getting back into the shape I had been in years earlier.

Exactly ninety days later, I had gone from a forty-four to a thirty-four inch waist. I'm living proof that you can get lean in twelve weeks at age forty. I'm about to share with you the details of how I did it and that's a big deal. Please join me now as we transform the world—one body at a time—starting with you. May this book forever change your life as it did mine.

Chapter 1

———⋙◆⋘———

Compare and Contrast

I will start by examining two of the top selling diet books that have sold in the tens of millions. From this point on, think of me as the messenger who weeds out fact from fiction. I know of no better way than to start with this approach.

There is a lot of truth to both *The South Beach Diet* and *The Abs Diet*, but there are issues that I cannot overlook. The twelve other diet books and programs I have read recently include: *Volumetrics, Enter The Zone, The Mediterranean Diet, The Atkins Diet, The Weight Watchers Diet, Skinny Bitch Diet, The Sugar Busters Diet, Eat This Not That Diet, Perfect Body Diet, The Superfoods Rx Diet, The Nutrisystem Diet,* and *The Jenny Craig Diet.*

These books and their teachings are generally redundant, containing typical calorie-reduction methods and some gimmick advice with few exceptions—my critiques would be repetitive. My biggest complaint is with the timing of the foods eaten and the types of foods recommended.

SOUTH BEACH DIET

The South Beach Diet is a diet plan created by a Florida based cardiologist Arthur Agatston. Agatston does a good job encouraging the increased consumption of good fats and good carbohydrates. The diet severely restricts carbohydrates in the first two weeks, before gradually re-introducing those with a low glycemic index—the ones that produce only small fluctuations in our blood glucose and insulin levels. He recommends swapping saturated fats for unsaturated ones and focuses on weight control. His book jumps from subject to subject in each chapter without a specific enough game plan that I would have liked to of seen. The timing and quantity of foods mentioned is how the Transform Diet will have answers that are more specific.

ARE DAIRY PRODUCTS GOOD FOR YOU?

Regardless of what studies or special interest groups are saying, here is the real scoop on what typically happens to most of us when we consume any form of dairy. Dr. Agatston is a fan of these products; I'm not.

If you truly want to get rid of your gut, you cannot consume dairy. There are compounds like lactose (milk sugar), even in skim milk that slow the metabolism. Fat-free isn't the issue. Sugar is—in most cases, the lactose in milk will prevent people from seeing a firm midsection.

Dr. Judyth Reichenberg-Ullman and Dr. Robert Ullman explain, "Many people confuse milk allergy and lactose intolerance, but they are two different conditions. Most of the world's population, excluding Northern Europeans and isolated groups in Northern India and Africa, are deficient in lactase, the enzyme needed to digest lactose, or milk sugar. These people, most notably African-Americans, Latin-Americans, and those of Mediterranean descent, develop gas, bloating, and intestinal cramping after eating dairy products."

Herbert Shelton, founder of the Hygienists, feels that any mucus-forming food, dairy being at the top of his list, is "poison." Harvey and Marilyn Diamond, authors of *Fit for Life*, proclaim emphatically that cow's milk is not fit for human consumption.

Of course, dairy products are filled with eight essential amino acids that are the building blocks of protein and dairy fat that contains conjugated linoleic acid, or CLA, is believed to aid in weight control. However, the slogan, "Milk does a body good!" is misleading—depending on how milk has been manipulated.

A big problem with most dairy is that you will develop a layer of water between the muscle and skin, leaving you wondering why the abs never surface—even after you're eating "clean" months down the road. Dairy products, as studies have shown, tend to hold water on the entire body. The "soft" look is where you're headed when you consume dairy products—even in small amounts.

My best advice is to watch your intake of all dairy for the first twelve weeks of starting this program. That being said, whey protein powder is a fantastic milk byproduct choice—as almost all of the lactose and fat have been removed in the process. The make-up is different and has very positive effects on the body. It should be a daily staple in your diet since your physique will harden up by doing so.

WHAT YOU NEED TO KNOW ABOUT FRUIT

I like what Dr. Agatston says about not juicing fruit. Insulin, a powerful hormone with extensive effects on metabolism, will spike drastically if the pulp is removed from the fruit. In fact, it's equivalent to stacking a multivitamin on a Mr. Goodbar.

In general, fruit can be detrimental if not eaten in moderation. Yes, there are key vitamins and minerals; however, they can be a serious enemy to the midsection for many of us—especially when eaten after lunch. This little known fact will supercharge your metabolism and let you move past the frustration of not seeing results quickly around the waistline.

The problem is fructose (fruit sugar). Six to twelve minutes after fructose enters your blood stream, it will be treated very much like sucrose (table sugar). The pulp will slow insulin—which is a good thing—but sugar eventually stores as fatty tissue if not burned off. It's a real killer. To the critics: I'm not condemning fruit, I'm simply telling you it can be trouble on an overweight body, especially if you are sedentary.

Fitness expert Gary Zeolla—who holds a nutritional science degree from Penn State—says, "Fruit is rightly promoted as being a very healthy food. Most fruits contain a high nutrient, phytonutrient, and antioxidant content, and there is a wealth of scientific evidence of the benefits of fruit consumption.

"The first argument is based on fruit's high sugar content. It is said that sugar of any sort is not good for you, even when it occurs naturally in fruit. Moreover, it is said that fruit today has higher sugar contents than yesteryear due to hybridization practices.

"All you have to do is compare the size and sweetness of an apple growing in the wild with an apple found at a grocery store. The grocery store apple most likely will be larger, have a brighter and more consistent red color, and most importantly, be sweeter. So basically, you'd have to eat two or three wild apples to get the same sugar content as one grocery store apple.

"However, this argument would not mean any fruit consumption is unhealthy. It would simply mean to consume fruit only in moderation. In other words, if one grocery store apple equals three wild apples, only eat one grocery store apple, not three."

Others agree; in the December 14, 2007, article in *ScienceDaily*, University of Florida researcher, Dr. Richard Johnson noted that, in relation to obesity, the type of fructose found in foods doesn't seem to matter. "The fructose in an apple is as problematic as the high-fructose corn syrup in soda. The apple is much more nutritious and contains far less sugar, but eating multiple apples in one sitting could send the body over the fructose edge."

In another University of Florida paper published in October 2007, the *American Journal of Clinical Nutrition*, Johnson and his collaborators tracked the rise of obesity and diseases such as diabetes with the rise in sugar consumption in fructose. The rates of hypertension, diabetes, and childhood obesity have risen steadily over the years.

Timing is another important factor to consider when eating fruit. Dr. Agatston likes fruit toward the evening, to prevent cravings. I believe that will be trouble for most of us. Depending on your body type and metabolism, you need to be careful of the time and amount of fruit you eat per day. On most physiques, eating complex carbohydrates after lunch—especially fruit— will not only disrupt, but destroy what you have been trying to accomplish. Even in my twenties, I noticed fruit caused belly fat—regardless of whether I was exercising daily or not.

Unless you have the body of an ectomorph—a very lean body that is forgiving of these types of carbohydrates and fructose—you're headed for trouble around the midsection, hips, and thighs. Fruit can be okay if eaten daily after twelve weeks on the Transform Diet—but definitely not after lunch and in moderation. Anything after 2:00 PM. and you will be going to bed while sugar is trying to metabolize, which obviously is not a good thing.

Again, timing is everything. I have trained men and women who insisted on eating fruit even after I told them not to. A month later, they came back saying how much body fat and weight they had gained, increasing dress and pant sizes.

After you have reached your goals and your metabolism has kicked into high gear, you might be able to take the plunge and eat fruit as freely as you wish. You will need to experiment on what works best for your body type.

SHOULD YOU EAT UNTIL YOU ARE SATISFIED?

The other big issues for me are the *"Two snacks in between meals"* and the *"Eat until you are satisfied"* theories. In my professional opinion, I disagree with Dr. Agatston's statements. The human body has a difficult time metabolizing anything over fifty grams of carbohydrates per meal (as I explain in Chapter 3). I used to eat until I was feeling satisfied—and I ended up weighing almost 260 pounds. As for snacking between meals, it usually doesn't work. Eating five solid meals will keep blood sugar balanced and your appetite suppressed.

Most Americans have no idea when they are satisfied. We eat larger portions than anyone in the world. We need guidance and structure. Most of us are thinking about the next meal even before it arrives, or worse, skipping meals because we overate during the previous meal.

Dr. Agatston explains that after spending two weeks on The South Beach Diet, "The cravings for sugars and starches are virtually gone, too." I'm not sure that's accurate. I think more specifically our bodies slow down the craving, but our minds still tell us not to let go. It's a battle that will go on for not only two weeks after starting a new diet, but as long as we live. Half of *The South Beach Diet*—like most of the others mentioned—is filled with recipes and testimonials.

THE ABS DIET

The Abs Diet is a nutritional diet created by *Men's Health* editor-in-chief David Zinczenko with the help of Ted Spiker.

The diet recommends six small meals spread throughout the day emphasizing the so-called *Twelve Power Foods*. The name of the diet is a little misleading. You're not guaranteed to end up with a six-pack in six weeks. The "Abs Diet" does not imply a focus on the abdominal muscles, but is an acronym representing the twelve power foods ("A" for almonds, etc.). The diet gives the readers one "free meal" per week, where they are allowed to eat anything they like.

The authors offer good advice about fats, proteins, and carbohydrates, but they expose themselves through their food choices and calorie-counting menu plans. There is no doubt that after reading their book and starting the program, you will lose weight. I believe they offered some intelligent and helpful tips that lead to a better body. Like the South Beach Diet, the Abs Diet leaves the reader with too many unanswered questions.

HOW OFTEN TO EAT?

A big problem I had with the Abs Diet is that it suggests eating foods with less than three hours between meals. There are side effects to this that will eventually lead to a slower metabolism and stored body fat.

Well-known clinical nutritionist Gregg Ladd advises, "Eat once every three hours. It takes that long for the last meal to move out of the stomach. If you eat too soon, the food you've already eaten will stop digesting, and the whole thing starts all over again. Food will actually remain in the intestines undigested for as long as two days."

Think how detrimental that would be on getting lean—it would make it very tough. It is also important to understand that going more than three hours without food is not recommended either. There is a very big problem with this habit; the human body begins to slow down to conserve energy—which will eventually be stored as fat—and burns calories less efficiently.

You could have the greatest meal plan ever, however if not eaten at the appropriate time, or in the wrong quantities, you will store fatty tissue. It's equivalent to having a great playbook in football without knowing when to run the play. You need a "coach" that understands timing and when to implement it. It's easily resolved when you eat clean (eating most foods in their natural state and staying away from junk food) every 3 hours. You need to be a stickler on this for the first 12 weeks, maintaining this as much as possible thereafter.

PROBLEMS WITH THE ABS DIET BREAKFAST PLANS

A typical breakfast meal plan they offer has to be a misprint. I have the utmost respect for David Zinczenko. I'm going to give him the benefit of the doubt, but I must tell you that what is recommended is not sound advice. The breakfast is *two tablespoons of peanut butter.*

Okay, I see where they are getting to the monounsaturated fat, but peanut butter is fifth on my monounsaturated fat list.

On *whole grain toast?*

You're starting to lose me, guys. The gluten in wheat toast is a killer for the love handles—and causes water retention—even if it is whole wheat. Whole wheat toast is very hard to metabolize for 75 percent of Americans.

With *two* slices of Canadian bacon?

You can't be serious. The body part from the pig's back is sweetened usually with sugar. And what about the sodium in bacon?

The Abs Diet also advices us to eat any cereal made with 3/4 cup of high-fiber, with a quarter-cup of Cap'n Crunch, with two tablespoons of almonds and 3/4 cup of 1 percent or fat-free milk. The almonds are a great choice of monounsaturated fat and will start the body fat process. Any high-fiber cereal will help in slowing the absorption of carbohydrates to speed the metabolism. Almonds and high fiber cereal are good choices, but they are counteracted with bad ones in the same meal.

What about the dairy products and processed cereal? Dairy contains compounds that cause gas, bloating, aching lower back, dry skin, clogged pours, sluggishness, and slowed metabolism. Processed cereal is also unforgiving for most of us—even in small amounts. It's just empty calories that slow the metabolism and holds water in the body.

Between the dairy and the Cap'n Crunch, I would have no choice but to look like the Michelin Man. I understand how throwing in a highly processed cereal can make the reader feel that it is easy, and it tastes good, and he or she will stick with the plan—but it just doesn't work. A quarter of a cup of anything processed kills the rest of the meal—especially when it's loaded with sugar. It counteracts fiber, destroys the diet, and adds unwanted body fat.

If this were my breakfast every day for six weeks, I would lose weight due to the lack of calories. However, my sodium intake would be off the charts and my waistline would feel like vanilla pudding.

Let me leave you with a final thought: with most of the books mentioned above, the basis is that consuming less food causes you to lose weight from a lack of caloric intake. Be aware that if you eat less but retain your current food profile, you will just construct a miniature version of your old self. Basically, less of the same will shrink you, but your proportion of muscle to body fat will stay the same. What is the end result? You look like your old self—just pounds lighter. I am convinced I can change that.

Chapter 2

<hr/>

Transform Diet vs. Dr. Mehmet Oz

I believe Oprah Winfrey has heard and seen it all. She is everything you could want in a leader. She is an icon. We all know she has at her fingertips the greatest minds, doctors, and trainers in the world. She gets advice from only the very best.

Regardless of her size, she always looks great, but I have a feeling she would like to be leaner. Her doctor, Dr. Mehmet Oz, is a cardiothoracic surgeon. He speaks regularly on XM Satellite Radio and is a regular guest on "The Oprah Winfrey Show."

To say that Dr. Oz is an expert on how the body breaks down food in an understatement. However, I would like to address some issues I have with his teachings. Dr. Oz's comments are taken directly from Oprah.com and *You: The Owner's Manual* by Memhet Oz and Michael Roizen.

Dr. Oz: Eat when you are hungry

Transform: With all due respect, this is not good advice. It is easy to upset the balance of blood sugar by skipping meals or waiting too long to eat. When blood sugar levels are normal, you feel calm yet energized. When you actually wait until you're hungry? Blood sugar levels will fall; your energy and mood will drop. You begin to store fat, and your metabolism will go into starvation mode. If you remember nothing else, know this; four hours from your last meal, your metabolism will go into starvation mode. The only time it should be shutting down like this is when you are asleep. The body is a finely tuned machine and needs to be treated as such. If not, you will look more like the Stay Puft Marshmallow Man.

Another problem with waiting until you are hungry to eat is losing control to the temptations of food that you are about to partake of. Food is like a drug. It will manipulate your brain and you will eat too much in one sitting. This, of course, stores more body fat. It's a recipe for obesity and I know that in the fight against fat, we need structure and consistency. This advice may work for some, but for the majority, you will never reach the goals.

Dr. Oz: Dr. Oz says that the way to get to where you want to be physically is to cut only one hundred calories per day

Transform: I have to disagree. I don't think calorie-counting works. I'm not sure an overweight person really cares about one hundred extra calories. No one really ever knows exactly how many calories they eat per day. I measure my foods depending on the meal—and still do not know the exact caloric intake in any particular meal. To truly know if I cut one hundred calories or not would be calorie counting. However, to be fair, it is important to measure food in many cases, at least in the beginning of the diet, as you need to look at carbohydrate consumption precisely. If Dr. Oz were simply to cut one hundred calories on a three-hundred-pound man, how much difference would it truly make?

Dr. Oz: Instead of focusing on the number on the scale, Dr. Oz says to focus on the number around your waist. "The ideal waistline for women is 32 ½ inches and 35 inches for a man—a goal that is achievable by everyone, no matter your age."

Transform: I agree about 70 percent with this statement. I'm trying to be more specific and detailed. I know thousands of women who would be devastated if they had a 32 ½-inch waist. It's a good number to work with, but it's too vague.

I believe everyone who eats, and has a pulse, can get below these figures. It's just a matter of time and what you're willing to do. To put the 32 ½-inch waist in perspective: a six foot one, 190-pound male who is in great shape is about 32–33 inches. I don't see how a five foot seven woman can want to have that size waist. She would have to weigh roughly 175 pounds. I don't believe that is a healthy weight for a woman regardless of age, especially considering men have more muscle than women do. To be fair, I believe Dr. Oz is trying to generalize by giving these measurements. For most, they can be obtained in a practical amount of time.

STOP COUNTING CARBOHYDRATES?

On Oprah.com, you can read this under a caption by Dr. Oz: **"Forget the fad diets. Stop counting carbohydrates."**

Dr. Oz obtained a joint MD and MBA degree from the University of Pennsylvania School of Medicine and the Wharton School in 1986. If Dr. Oz truly believes counting carbohydrates is not necessary, this is probably why: the school of thought at that time was the American Heart Association's recommendation of a high-carbohydrate, low fat diet. Unfortunately for Dr. Oz, he graduated one year before maybe one of the greatest discoveries in the twentieth century—the genetic mystery regarding how carbohydrates affect insulin.

THE PROFOUND FINDINGS AT STANFORD UNIVERSITY

In 1987, one year after Dr. Oz graduated from college, Stanford University researcher Gerald Reaven, discovered the genetic mystery regarding insulin surge with carbohydrates, and that counting carbohydrates is fundamentally necessary.

Reaven pointed out that 25 percent of the population had no response to carbohydrates. This meant they could eat all their hearts desired. He also found 25 percent of the population at the opposite end of the spectrum to have a significant response to carbohydrates and stored significant amounts of body fat. He concluded that the rest of us fit between the two extremes.

The study showed that the middle 50 percent of the population, have a moderately elevated response to carbohydrates, and if we are not careful, we store that "spillage" of carbohydrates as fat. Reaven is now professor of medicine at Stanford University. He served as director of the Division of Endocrinology and Metabolism. He is considered one of the greatest minds in the world, and understands insulin and its role on carbohydrates better than anyone.

THE LATEST RESEARCH ON CARBOHYDRATES

- **Phil Maffetone, PhD, one of the world's foremost experts in exercise physiology, athletic training, and coaching says this:** "Today's school of thought on high-carbohydrate, low-fat diets is quickly changing, as people begin to realize that even after consistently working out, they are not losing body fat. Since most carbohydrates contain little or no fat, you may not think that carbohydrates can add to your fat stores. Yet, at least 40 percent of the carbohydrates you eat are stored as fat."

- "Consuming too many carbohydrates—even fat-free—can actually make you fat. That's because of the way your body stores and uses the end product of the carbohydrates you consume. Carbohydrates, whether they are in the form of pastas or chocolate cake, turn into glucose once they enter the bloodstream. Sugar is sugar—the body doesn't discriminate. So, if you consume excess amounts of carbohydrates, your blood sugar levels increase, triggering your pancreas to release insulin. Insulin controls where in the body blood sugar is stored. Some is used for energy, and some is stored in the muscles as glycogen (the stored form of sugar)."

- **Gary Taubes, American science writer:** Taubes has won the Science in Society Award of the National Association of Science Writers three times and was awarded an MIT Knight Science "Journalism Federation grant" for 1996–97. Taubes studied applied physics at Harvard and aerospace engineering at Stanford.

- After receiving a master's degree in journalism at Columbia University in 1981, Taubes joined *Discover* as a staff reporter in 1982. Since then, he has written numerous articles for *Discover, Science*, and other magazines. Originally focusing on physics issues, his interests have more recently turned to medicine and nutrition.

- "After re-reading years of scientific research, science has just gotten it wrong: it's not fat that is making Americans fat, it is the base of the food pyramid, the complex carbohydrates, such as bread, pasta, and potatoes. Carbs spike insulin. Insulin creates sugar. And sugar packs on the pounds."

- *The New England Journal of Medicine*: **March 2007 report:** "Participants who successfully followed low-carbohydrate plans for six months lost more weight than those who ate low-fat or high carbohydrate diet."

- **Barry Sears, PhD, biochemist:** One of the world's leading medical researchers on the hormonal effects of food says, "The consumption of carbohydrates such as pasta and bread can cause a sharp spike in insulin production, and if this happens chronically, we start to gain weight. This leads to insulin resistance and eventually results in a dangerous condition known as 'silent inflammation.' Carbohydrates are the reason you are fat."

- **Barry Groves, PhD, world-renowned researcher and author wrote in 2007,** "Carbs and carbs alone, not fat, increase body weight. It doesn't matter whether the carbohydrates are from sugar, bread, or fruit: They're all rapidly digested and quickly converted to blood glucose."

- "A short time after a carb-rich meal, the glucose in your bloodstream rises rapidly, and your pancreas produces a large amount of insulin to take the excess glucose out. Just as eating fat doesn't raise blood glucose; it doesn't raise insulin levels either. This is important because insulin is the hormone responsible for body fat storage. Because fats do not elicit an insulin response, they cannot be stored as body fat. Insulin takes glucose out of the bloodstream. It is converted first into a starch called glycogen, which is stored in the liver and in muscles. But the body can store only a limited amount of glycogen, so the excess glucose is stored as body fat. This is the process of putting on weight."

- "When your blood glucose level returns to normal, after about ninety minutes, the insulin level in your bloodstream is still near maximum. As a result, the insulin continues to stack glucose away in the form of fat. Ultimately, the level of glucose in your blood falls below normal, and you feel hungry again. So, you have a snack of more carbohydrates, and the whole process starts over again. You're getting fatter, but feeling hungry at the same time. Ultimately, insulin resistance caused by continually high insulin levels in your bloodstream impairs your ability to switch on a satiety center in the brain. You enter a vicious cycle of continuous weight gain combined with hunger."

- **In March 2008, the University of Iowa's entire healthcare system** said, "Carbohydrates are the great balancing act."

- **In a 2007 Harvard University study, David Ludwig** found that sixty-four overweight adolescents who were told to eat lower-glycemic-index foods lost an average of four pounds, while forty-three overweight adolescents who were told to make modest cuts in calories and fat gained three pounds. "Carbohydrates definitely play a role in weight gain."

- **Stanford University, John W. Farquhar, MD professor of Medicine and Health Research & Policy says**, "Too many carbohydrates will raise triglycerides, lower HDL cholesterol, and make LDL small and dense, all of which raises the risk of heart disease."

- **UCLA researchers, April 1, 2007:** "Americans are getting fatter. In fact, more than 60 percent are overweight and 18 million have Type 2 diabetes. It's an epidemic that's becoming more of a problem with each passing year. Now, a new discovery could help you shed those dangerous pounds and live a healthier life. Pastas ... breads ... cereals ... We know them well. And doctors say it's carbohydrates like these that are making us fat.

The problem is that starches are broken down immediately into sugars. When starch breaks down into sugar, it stays in the bloodstream, but is eventually stored as fat."

- **Chris Aceto, world-renowned nutritionist:** "You also have to account for ratios of carbohydrates, protein, and fat. Then there's meal frequency too: from real-world results, we know you put down more muscle mass from five or six meals a day than from three meals a day. There are more things involved than just calories."

- **Clinical nutritionist Jay Robb**: "From the late 1970s until around the mid-1990s, America was predominantly following a high-carbohydrate, low-fat diet that was supposed to make fat melt away like magic. Unfortunately, during that time period, Americans became fatter than ever. Why? Because excessive consumption of high-carbohydrate foods stimulates the release of a hormone called insulin. It has four primary jobs: 1) to stop you from burning fat; 2) to allow you to burn glucose as energy; 3) to help you store excess glucose as glycogen (muscle starch for later use); and 4) to convert excess blood sugar into fat ... *body fat*! So, when America cut calories on a low-fat, high-carbohydrate diet, it was a disaster that ended up making Americans fatter than ever! And basically America's 'weight problem' was primarily caused by the over consumption of carbohydrates."

- **Greg Joujon-Roche, personal trainer to the stars**. He trained Brad Pitt for *Troy*, Tobey Maguire for *Spider-Man*, Demi Moore for *G.I. Jane*, just to name a few. "I love carbs—starch and sugar—but I've learned to be very moderate in my consumption of them. They're too much like a drug. They sprint into your bloodstream, spike up your blood sugar and insulin, and then leave you longing for more."

THE FINAL WORD

To say that counting carbohydrates is a "fad diet" is ridiculous. We know that being in a state of ketosis (less than fifty grams of carbohydrates per day, according to The Atkins Diet) burns body fat faster than any program. It's proven with the best doctors in the world, and on people every day, as well as me. We also know that it's not completely safe.

The trick is to be just above ketosis (see Chapter 3), through carbohydrate intake, creating an avenue for the body to metabolize food and burn body fat. It's the amount and timing of carbohydrates like pasta, breads, and cereals that have turned America fat.

Dr. Oz's sole purpose is to make America a healthier place. He does a fantastic job at this. He is looking for overall health, removing simple carbohydrates from the diet and replacing them with complex carbohydrates. Like most doctors I know, he is not overly concerned with external issues like hardening of the body or tightening of the skin. His basis is eating correctly to fight heart disease and making us internally healthy. The Transform Diet is specifically about carbohydrate, protein, and fat intake. Although we share common goals, we are worlds apart on how to get there.

I'm convinced that if Ms. Oprah Winfrey ate three meals of starch carbohydrates (the ones I have laid out in Chapter 8) not exceeding one hundred grams of carbohydrates in her first three settings, then switched to fibrous carbohydrates for the remaining two, eating every three hours, it would change her body once and for all. She would see drastic results.

Chapter 3

<hr/>

Carbohydrates

In order for you to really understand why and how this diet is going to work, you need to know the facts. I will try to keep it as simple as I can—not giving you my opinion but what has been researched by the top doctors, dieticians, biochemists, cardiologists, and nutritional experts in the world.

WHAT ARE CARBOHYDRATES?

Carbohydrates are eaten in two forms: simple and complex. Simple carbohydrates are smaller molecules of sugar unlike the long chains in starch. They are digested quickly because the individual sugars are ready to be absorbed immediately since digestive enzymes have easy access to these bonds. In order to transform, these carbohydrates are the ones you need to consistently avoid.

Examples of simple carbohydrates are corn syrup, fruit juice, candy, most breads and other baked goods made with white flour, soda, table sugar, and most packaged cereals.

Complex carbohydrates are simply sugars bonded together to form a chain. Digestive enzymes have to work much harder to access the bonds to break the chain into individual sugars for absorption through the intestines. This is a good thing—the harder it is for the body to break carbohydrates down into sugar, the faster your metabolism, and the tighter your physique.

Complex carbohydrates are the ones you should be eating in most of your meals. The slow absorption of sugars provides us with a steady supply of energy and limits the amount of sugar converted into fat and stored. Lettuce, spinach, asparagus, broccoli, onions, apples, strawberries, brown rice, oatmeal, and rye are some examples of complex carbohydrates. Although these are complex carbohydrates, don't assume you can eat them freely as the timing and quantity must be monitored carefully.

The two types of carbohydrates I want you to focus on are *starch* and *fibrous*. Examples of *starch carbohydrates* are rice, potatoes, pasta, fruit, and cereals along with some others. Examples of *fibrous carbohydrates* are lettuce, spinach, broccoli, onions, tomatoes, and cucumbers. Basically, they are leafy greens and mostly vegetables. It is important to notice that most fruits are starch carbohydrates and most vegetables are fibrous carbohydrates. What does that tell us? It tells us that there is a big difference between the two types of carbohydrates when it comes to calories, and the amount of carbohydrates in each.

Starch carbohydrates should only be eaten up until lunch, as they are loaded with many calories and convert to fat if not burned off. Fibrous carbohydrates can be eaten in high quantities, at any time day or night. In fact, an entire bag of spinach leaves has a total of twelve grams of carbohydrates—whereas one large banana has thirty-nine grams of carbohydrates. Also, the sugar content between the two is at opposite ends of the spectrum. Keep this in mind as you continue to read. Knowing this fact will change your body indefinitely.

THE SCIENCE OF CARBOHYDRATES

It is a known fact that we need a certain amount of carbohydrates to feed our brains and bodies. The body requires a continual intake of carbohydrates to feed the brain, which uses glucose (a sugar) to get its primary source of energy. It is critical to understand that any carbohydrates not used by the body will be stored in the form of glycogen (glucose molecules linked together).

World-renowned biochemist Dr. Barry Sears says, "The body has two storage sites for glycogen: the liver and the muscles. The glycogen stored in the muscles is inaccessible to the brain. Only the glycogen stored in the liver can be broken down and sent back to the bloodstream as to maintain adequate blood sugar levels for proper brain function."

Sears also states, "Once the glycogen levels are filled in both the liver and muscles, excess carbohydrates have just one fate, to be converted into fat and stored in the adipose, that is, fatty, tissue."

It is these very facts we will go after on the Transform Diet. It's the key to getting you lean, and it's this very point that will change your body makeup forever.

The human body is a like a machine or car engine, it needs "fuel." One major difference is our "gas tank" goes empty about every three hours and—if you don't "refill it"—it begins to shut down. Here is a fact that every nutritional source I can find agrees with about the breakdown of carbohydrates.

Iowa State University's department of health: "A well-nourished adult can store approximately five hundred grams or two thousand kcal of carbohydrates. Of this, approximately four hundred grams are stored as muscle glycogen, 90–110 grams as liver glycogen, and two to three grams circulate in the blood as glucose. When the body needs more glucose than is available in the bloodstream to support energy demands, glycogen stores are used to raise blood glucose levels. However, it is important to note that the glycogen stored in muscle is used directly by that muscle during exercise, it cannot borrow glycogen from other resting muscles."

The critical question now becomes "How many carbohydrates can I eat every three hours to maximize both liver and muscle glycogen levels without spilling over to fat?" If the experts tell us we store a maximum of four hundred grams as muscle glycogen and another one hundred as liver glycogen, we know anything above this will be converted into fat, unless it's burned off through exercise. There is no gray area when it comes to understanding that excess carbohydrates do store as fat.

In fact, Dr. Barry Sears says, "The question no one has bothered to ask until now is this: What happens when you eat too many carbohydrates? Whether it's being stored in the liver or the muscles, the total storage capacity of the body for carbohydrates is really quite limited. If you're an average person, you can store about three hundred to four hundred grams of carbohydrates in your muscles. In the liver, where carbohydrates are accessible for glucose conversion, you can store only about sixty to ninety grams."

So, what if you are not "average"? Then what? For starters, the powerful hormone leptin is produced by fat cells. It ignites best when eating moderate to low amount of carbs per day—as I explain shortly—then switching to a high-carb meal. Secondly, I would play it safe and think of yourself as having a slow metabolism and not being "average."

For 30 percent of you, three hundred grams per day may be the answer. For the majority of you, this number is still too high and you will not see the results you are looking for if you consume that many carbohydrates over a twelve-hour period. Depending on the amount of skeletal muscle—as well as your amount of daily exercise—will determine whether that number can rise or fall. Don't take a chance for the first twelve weeks and guess. I personally have seen two hundred grams being the largest number in nearly 70 percent of all people I have trained and put on diets over the past ten years—at least for the first twelve weeks. Dr. Sears as well as Iowa State are generalizing. I'm trying to be very specific.

Here is how it works:

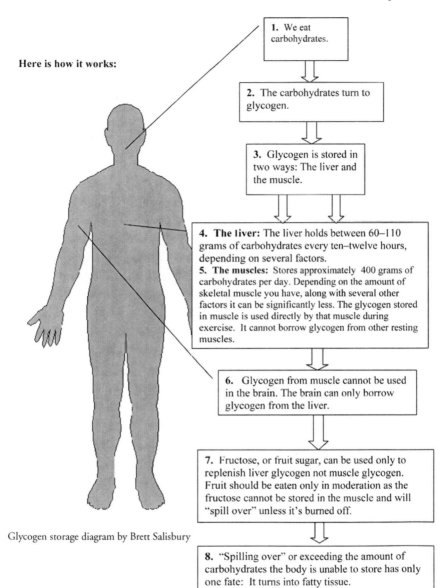

1. We eat carbohydrates.

2. The carbohydrates turn to glycogen.

3. Glycogen is stored in two ways: The liver and the muscle.

4. The liver: The liver holds between 60–110 grams of carbohydrates every ten–twelve hours, depending on several factors.

5. The muscles: Stores approximately 400 grams of carbohydrates per day. Depending on the amount of skeletal muscle you have, along with several other factors it can be significantly less. The glycogen stored in muscle is used directly by that muscle during exercise. It cannot borrow glycogen from other resting muscles.

6. Glycogen from muscle cannot be used in the brain. The brain can only borrow glycogen from the liver.

7. Fructose, or fruit sugar, can be used only to replenish liver glycogen not muscle glycogen. Fruit should be eaten only in moderation as the fructose cannot be stored in the muscle and will "spill over" unless it's burned off.

8. "Spilling over" or exceeding the amount of carbohydrates the body is unable to store has only one fate: It turns into fatty tissue.

Glycogen storage diagram by Brett Salisbury

WHAT HAPPENS WHEN I "SPILL OVER" TO CREATE FATTY TISSUE?

"Fat cells are surprisingly complicated," says Dr. David Heber, professor of medicine at the UCLA Geffen School of Medicine and director of the UCLA Center for Human Nutrition. "They're more than a bag of fat."

Humans have about 40 billion fat cells in their body, and each cell contains an oily substance called lipids. An obese person has at least two to three times that. And obese people have much larger fat cells than lean ones. If a person keeps overeating, fat cells grow and grow, looking as if they are about to explode. Those lipids can expand up to about one thousand times their original size. In some people, each cell can end up swelling to a diameter of three hundred microns—almost big enough to see with the naked eye. The fat we see on ourselves are multiple fat cells combined together. When they reach the limit, they don't divide; they send out a signal to nearby immature cells to start dividing to produce more fat cells. Recent research tells us that unlike red and white blood cells, fat cells do not have the capability of dissolving and leaving the body. They remain for life.

Once the fat is burned from the cell, they become microscopic in size. So for each day you continue to expand the fat cells in your body, it becomes two and three times harder to lose those lipids.

According to *Medical News Today*: "Scientists used to think body fat was pretty much inert, just an oily storage compartment. But in the past decade, research has shown that fat cells are chemical factories and that body fat is potent stuff: a highly active tissue that secretes hormones and other substances with profound and sometimes harmful effects on metabolism, weight, and overall health."

"In recent years, biologists have begun calling fat an 'endocrine organ,' comparing it to glands such as the thyroid and pituitary, which also release hormones straight into the bloodstream. But those glands cannot grow nearly as much as fat, which has a seemingly infinite capacity to make more of itself. Too much body fat can act like a poison, spewing out substances that contribute to diabetes, heart disease, high blood pressure, stroke, and other illnesses, including some cancers. The best way to get rid of visceral fat (abdominal fat) and shrink fat cells all at once is diet and exercise."

WHEN AND HOW TO EAT CARBOHYDRATES

Eat specific carbohydrates every three hours. This way you will not have a dip in blood sugar, and you will keep your metabolism burning at 100 percent. We need to eat just enough to feed the muscle and liver and not spill to store fat. We also want to stay out of the controversial method of ketosis *(Dr. Atkins Diet)*. Dr. Atkins keeps carbohydrates below the recommended levels so your body has no choice but to burn fat. It works, but his levels dip below fifty grams of carbohydrates per day—which affect liver glycogen levels and your brain.

The dreadful outcome of eating too many carbohydrates puts a tremendous toll on the metabolism, especially combined with other foods. So, the *"Eat until you're satisfied"* theory (*South Beach Diet*), or *"Pick and choose what you want, when you want carbohydrate"* theory *(Abs Diet)* as evidence shows, are inaccurate. Forget the latest fad diet or what is "hot" at the moment. The fact is that any diet plan keeping you just above ketosis works best on the most stubborn physique.

Let's look at what a typical male and female require for carbohydrate intake every day and specifically every three hours.

If an adult male eats fifty grams of carbohydrates per meal, three times per day, while eating around twenty grams of fibrous carbs in the remaining two meals, he would get roughly 170 grams of carbohydrates. Of the 170, he would then need around ninety of those carbohydrates to use as liver glycogen, which the muscle cannot borrow from. I highly recommend following this to the T if you want drastic results.

An adult male would need around 170 carbohydrates per day to stay full and not spill over to fat, while giving his brain all the energy it could ever use. This will have met the liver glycogen requirements, regardless of your current size. The number differs slightly with each individual based on age, sex, race, activity levels, skeletal muscle, and a few other factors. Realizing every human being is different, this amount of carbohydrates can go slightly up or down—depending on what you want to weigh. However, I wouldn't exceed two hundred grams for the first twelve weeks—no matter how big you currently are. I break down every meal completely in Chapter 8.

The female should try not exceed 125 grams of carbohydrates per day. This would be approximately twenty-five grams or less of carbohydrates per meal. Remember in both scenarios you are eating to the weight you want to be, not your current weight. For example, if you want to weigh 125 pounds and you currently weigh 185 pounds, I recommend eating one gram of carbohydrates per pound of future body weight. You would then eat 125 grams of specific carbohydrates per day. I have news for you. If you eat like this daily for twelve weeks—you will transform. Period.

In the movie *300*, this is how they lived and changed their bodies so drastically in three months. The actors were plain and simply ripped to the bone and so internally healthy their scores were off the charts. In fact, a rumor was that they were enhanced by special effects to give the achieved look because they looked so good on screen. The truth is they ate how I have stated above and worked out vigorously for twelve weeks—transforming from head to toe.

The trainer for *300* was Mark Twight. He pushed these actors to the limit. Had they simply gone into the weight room to train and not eaten specific carbohydrates at the appropriate times, they would have never looked like this. The greatest part is that the actors and actresses were not in great shape before the filming and most of them were pushing forty.

The Leptin Hormone trick

Here is the part you will love—the part you rarely read about in any diet book and the one you will be forever grateful for. It is how to release the hormone *leptin* to change and shock your metabolism in such a way that you *need* to eat a cheat meal, once a week after the fourth week—as it forces you to burn calories at a higher rate and changes your metabolic rate. It's essential and its part of the bigger picture.

Leptin itself was discovered in 1994 by Jeffrey M. Friedman and colleagues at Rockefeller University. Leptin is the Greek word for thin. Human leptin is a protein of 167 amino acids. It is manufactured in fat cells and the level of leptin circulating in the body is directly proportional to the total amount of fat in the body. The higher the leptin levels on a daily basis, the fatter you are.

Leptin controls your hunger, metabolism, and appetite. Researchers at the University of Wisconsin found that mice with low leptin levels had a faster metabolism and were able to burn fat faster than animals with high levels. Leptin basically tells the brain how much fat is in the body, and the body responds as such. Remember misery loves company. This means your existing fat is literally calling out for more fat.

Here is how the leptin trick works: if you stay in the carbohydrate ratios described above, your leptin level, body fat, and glycogen in your muscle drop significantly in about four weeks. As this happens, leptin begins to decline since it goes hand in hand with your fat. When levels drop, the body will protect itself and hit a sticking point in weight and metabolism. Leptin is extra sensitive to glucose, so eating a cheat meal; basically, any high carbohydrate meal (I usually can eat an entire pizza in one sitting) causes a surge in leptin that speeds your metabolism beyond what it has been weeks prior. Let me be perfectly clear, leptin doesn't affect fat loss. The effects of leptin do.

UCLA exercise physiologist Lyle McDonald explained: "I'd say leptin may be one of, if not *the* most important hormone when it comes to dieting and fat loss. I could literally talk about it all day, but I'll spare you the pain. See, during a diet, leptin drops much faster than body fat percentage. After seven days on a diet, leptin may be down by 50 percent from normal. Of course, you haven't lost 50 percent of your body fat. After that, leptin will continue to go down along with body fat percentage. It's the drop in leptin that 'tells' your brain: 'Hey, we're starving, shut the system down.' One researcher (in a 1998 paper) made an oblique reference to my idea that maintaining leptin levels on a diet might be more important. But nobody followed it up until a few months ago."

Fitness expert Shannon Clark said, "Leptin is highly responsive to glucose metabolism so when doing a 're-feed,' you will benefit much more if the majority of your excess calories are coming from good sources of carbohydrates that will turn into glucose. When done this way, leptin levels will show a significant rise over if you had eaten a surplus of calories coming from more protein, fat, or fructose."

Jeffrey Friedman, MD, PhD, professor at the Rockefeller University and an associate investigator with Howard Hughes Medical Institute says, "We found the amount of leptin highly correlates to how much fat is stored in the body, with greater levels found in individuals with more fat and reduced levels in those who dieted."

The Final World

The human body is very smart; it continually wants to adapt. This is where a new surge of leptin from a cheat meal doesn't allow the body to have a sticking point with its release. It's why you will want to pay the price in the first four weeks you started the Transform Diet, and not eat a cheat meal. The nice part is that research has shown that a surge of leptin in the body for a short period of time changes things drastically for the better. Typically, we see that another cheat meal, a week later, needs to be eaten to again trick the body, causing an increase in calories burned per hour.

After the fourth week, have one cheat meal to send a surge of leptin as this is the body's response to glucose. By doing this, your metabolism will drastically speed up. You will then eat clean for another six days allowing leptin to drop again. On the seventh day each week forward, you will partake of the cheat meal. This cycle needs to be continued for life as you will lose extreme levels of body fat and keep your metabolism roaring. The catch is if you don't remove excess carbohydrates from the diet for four weeks, the levels remain elevated and there will be no surge.

Chapter 4

$\Longleftarrow\!\!\!\!\Longrightarrow\!\!\!\bullet\!\!\Diamond\!\!\bullet\!\!\Longleftarrow\!\!\!\!\Longrightarrow$

Protein and Fats

PROTEIN

Like carbohydrates, the amount of protein per pound of body weight has become very controversial. However, the exciting news is that the latest research has proved to be spot on. I wanted to clear up any misunderstandings that may still linger. I am convinced that after reading this chapter, you will no longer have any doubts about what you need to do.

Proteins are appropriately named. The word protein is of Greek derivation and means "of first importance." Proteins are composed of chemical compounds called amino acids. Amino acids are usually called "the building blocks of protein," because they are combined to form the thousands of proteins in the human body.

Protein is the basis for all life on earth. Other than water, it is the most plentiful substance in our body. In each of our cells, protein is the main structural ingredient. Our immune system is primarily protein.

There are twenty amino acids, but only nine are considered essential to humans. Essential amino acids are necessary for normal growth and development and must be provided in the diet. Foods that primarily consist of protein are red meat, chicken, fish, turkey, pork, eggs, dairy products, soy, and whey (derivative of cow milk) as well as some others.

WHY IS PROTEIN CRUCIAL?

Eating too much or too little can create havoc on your body. According to nutritionist Greg Ladd, "Protein regulates insulin levels. When fewer than twenty grams of protein are consumed at breakfast, fat is stored for energy, not broken down. Hypoglycemia (low blood sugar) all day long is the result."

Eating too little protein also starts the condition called protein malnutrition, which includes loss of muscle, a weakened immune system, hair loss, increased body fat, slow metabolism, and negative nitrogen balance.

The highly regarded Ruth A. Roth, MS, RD and Carolynn E. Townsend, BA, say, "When people are unable to obtain an adequate supply of protein for an extended period of time, muscle wasting will occur and arms and legs will become very thin. At the same time, albumin (protein in blood plasma) deficiency will cause edema, which results in an extremely swollen appearance. People may lose appetite, strength, and weight, and wounds may heal very slowly. Patients suffering from edema become lethargic and depressed."

This is not a problem only with starving children in Africa. It's happening everyday in the United States of America. Roth and Townsend continue, "People following a vegetarian or vegan diet are susceptible. It is essential that people following vegetarian diets, especially vegans, carefully calculate the types and amount of protein in their diets so as to avoid protein deficiency."

THE PROBLEM WITH KETOSIS

Daily protein intake is critical and crucial with each meal. Since the 1970s, we have known that high-protein, low-carbohydrate diets are the fastest way to lose weight. We have also known that dropping carbohydrates below fifty grams usually puts the body in a state known as ketosis. Ketosis is simply when you have insufficient carbohydrates stored in the liver to meet the requirements of the body and the brain. Once the carbohydrate is used, which can take less than twenty-four hours; the body will turn to fat and muscle for energy.

Nutritional science expert Dr. Michael R. Eades says, "If you're starving, glucose can really come from only one place and that is from the protein reservoir: muscle. A little can come from stored fat, but not from the fatty acids themselves. Although glucose can be converted to fat, the reaction can't go the other way. Thus, a starving person can get a little glucose from the fat that is released from the fat cells, but not nearly enough. The lion's share has to come from muscle that breaks down into amino acids, several of which can be converted by the liver into glucose."

It's this chemistry of the body that no one can deny. It's why the Atkins diet works above all others for immediate weight loss. No diet book—including mine—can claim otherwise. Unfortunately, the process of converting fat into energy gets short-circuited on a carbohydrate diet this low. Atkins should have probably called this the ketogenic diet.

The result is that your cells manufacture abnormal biochemicals called ketone bodies. It's the side effect you don't want. In this state, the body will go through increased urination to try to rid the body of these ketones. You will lose weight and shrink the fat cells. You will also dip eventually into lean muscle regardless of protein intake, due to the lack of carbohydrates. It will ultimately affect your pH balance, which is not what you want to do.

Dr. Amy Joy Lanou, director of the Physicians Committee for Responsible Medicine in America, was quick to point out the health dangers of the Atkins diet. "A Harvard study published earlier this year in the Annals of Internal Medicine showed that high-protein diets may cause permanent loss of kidney function in anyone with reduced kidney function. Other studies have shown that meat-heavy diets significantly increase one's risk of colon cancer and osteoporosis."

Brigid McKevith, a nutrition scientist at the British Nutrition Foundation, said, "There could be difficulties for people who have an underlying problem with their kidneys or liver, because it would be putting more strain on those organs, and problems in terms of heart disease too, as it's a diet very low in fruits and vegetables. Also, it's very low in fiber, so in terms of digestive health, it's not in keeping with our fiber and complex carbohydrate recommendations."

Three major problems I have with the ketogenic diet (I have lived in this state). The first sounds more like a hygiene problem. It's called "halitosis-ketone breath." In a ketogenic state, the body needs energy, so it starts breaking down fat to produce energy. So far, so good.

The problem is that when the human body begins to break down fat, it releases a chemical in the body that causes bad breath. The chemical released is a ketone. Ketones are a byproduct or waste product from when your body burns stored fat for energy. Too many ketones from no carbohydrates results in halitosis. Halitosis means that whomever you are standing next to needs a gas mask. It is nasty.

The second problem is that when the brain gets less than fifty grams of carbohydrates per day over a three-day period, many people complain of blurred vision and the inability to think straight. It's happened to me. The brain is in need of glucose, which is the primary culprit.

What happens then? Even though glucose can be made out of protein, the protein that is keeping your muscles intact is now being used for energy, which eventually leads the muscle to be used as energy, starting a dreadful and vicious cycle. Can you imagine your body actually eating muscle for energy?

Lack of muscle means slower metabolism. Slower metabolism means stored body fat. Basically, ketones replace glucose. It's not what was ever intended for the body. There is no question you will lose significant amounts of weight and some body fat, but what are the long-term effects?

I have great respect for clinical nutritionist Jay Robb (he has his own protein powder line). He was a pioneer in nutrition, who considered himself a "human laboratory." In the early 1990s and before the mainstream, he figured out just what ketosis meant. I think he says it best in his own words:

"Ketosis is a radical fat burning state, but it is not (in my opinion) the best way to burn fat for a lifetime. Having worked with thousands of individuals in my twenty+ year career as a fitness professional, consultant, personal trainer, nutritional counselor, and gym owner, ketosis is great for burning fat for only very short periods of time. Eventually, if a person stays in ketosis, the body can get nervous because it believes you are starving, due to an extremely low carbohydrate intake. And when the body gets nervous about starving, many times its first reaction is to shut down your metabolism. And a lowered metabolism spells disaster.

"Without glycogen reserves, the body is assuming that food is scarce, so it shuts down to preserve your life in case of famine. This is easily detected by taking your body temperature during the day. Your temperature should be around 98.6 degrees Fahrenheit if your metabolism is up to speed.

"If your body believes you are starving either through low-calorie, low-fat, low-carb, or low-protein intake (or all of the previous), then it shuts down and your body temperature reflects this by dropping. The longer you diet, the lower your temperature (metabolism) may plunge. Midday readings of 96 or 97 degrees can often mean your metabolism is in super-slow motion and will force your body to hang on to all of its fat reserves. And if your metabolism stays low, you may even start to gain weight on low calorie meals. So now you see the problem unveiled."

What looks good in the beginning of ketosis is rapid weight loss due to the water being flushed out, as well as some fat. Anyone that has ever tried the Atkins Diet usually loses more weight in a two week period that any other. It makes complete sense. As for the daily consumption of sausage, bacon, and red meat at every meal, the saturated fat intake is a recipe for heart disease.

Another issue with this diet is the high amount of protein eaten in one meal. Having no carbohydrate in any meal causes overeating of proteins and saturated fats, forcing your kidneys to do a lot of work in breaking down the food, while raising your bad cholesterol to new heights and lowering your good cholesterol. Too much protein in one meal also causes insulin levels to increase, despite the help of fiber or fat. Exceeding fifty grams of protein per meal also puts added stress on the kidneys as well as other organs. A huge problem is that most people on this particular diet don't count the grams of protein in each meal; they simply eat away and hope that it all works out in the end.

THE PROTEIN CONTROVERSY

Here is the controversy. The USDA would like us to eat 0.36 grams of protein per pound of body weight. With all due respect, this recommendation is a joke. People on low-protein diets complain of having no real definition, while lacking overall muscle hardness throughout the body. A metabolism on this kind of diet is slow, lethargic, weak, and unable to heal properly as well as suffering from a negative nitrogen balance. I believe, like every other professional in this business, the USDA's findings are outdated and need to be reformed.

Dr. Anne Louise Gittleman, PhD, on protein intake: "As far as exact amounts are concerned, the jury is still out. For years, I have concurred with the Food and Nutrition Board of the National Research Council, which recommends seventy grams of protein for adult men and fifty-eight grams for women. To me, these numbers represent the bare minimum requirements, not the amounts for optimal health. The best way to figure out what works for you is by trial and error."

Dr. Atkins' new diet revolution is now 1.09 grams of protein per pound of body weight. Too much protein causes acidity in the body; it also causes major stress on the liver and kidneys. Unless you are a heavy strength trainer, bodybuilder, or professional athlete, steer clear of this recommendation.

THE FINAL ANSWER ON PROTEIN INTAKE

Dr. Peter Lemon is one of the world's leading researchers on protein requirements. He and a team of experts from Kent State University and McMaster University studied a group of twelve male subjects during two months of resistance training. They found that a protein intake of eighty-one grams per day, for a 180-pound male results in a negative nitrogen balance. The grams of protein came to 0.45 grams per pound of body weight. Still higher than the USDA, but not good enough.

Nitrogen balance is a measure of protein metabolism. A negative nitrogen balance indicates that the protein needs of the body are not being met. Over time, this may lead a person to burn his or her own muscle for energy, resulting in a series of catastrophic events, including slowed metabolism.

However, Dr Lemon also reported that at higher protein intakes, which works out at 214 grams for a 180-pound male. The nitrogen balance appeared to plateau and he and his team consider it "protein overload." The protein was at 1.19 grams per pound of body weight. Close to the Atkins Diet, but overkill.

Based on these findings, Dr. Lemon suggests for a 180-pound male, a protein intake of between 131 grams and 139 grams per day. Dr. Lemon's findings suggests 0.73 grams of protein per pound of body weight, which concurs precisely with other breakthrough information you are about to read.

CONCLUSIVE EVIDENCE

Jim Barlow, editor of *Life Science,* recently wrote: "As nutrition experts debate the ideal combination of protein, carbohydrates, and fat that people should eat, new research explains for the first time how and why a moderately high-protein diet may be the best for losing weight. The new findings suggest that eating more high-quality protein will increase the amount of leucine, an amino acid, in the diet, helping a person maintain muscle mass and reduce body fat during weight loss. Maintaining muscle during weight loss efforts is essential because it helps the body burn more calories."

The new research was led by Donald K. Layman, professor of nutrition in the department of food science and human nutrition at the University of Illinois at Urbana-Champaign. Here is what we know: leucine is universally regarded as the most potent BCAA (branched chain amino acid) for muscle growth. Don't get turned off by that. It's good for both the lean and overweight person. Leucine is a powerful activator of protein synthesis and, as Dr. Layman discovered, it also helps prevent muscle tissue breakdown and burns body fat.

"There's an additive, interactive effect when a protein-rich diet is combined with exercise. The two work together to correct body composition; dieters lose more weight, and they lose fat, not muscle. A higher-carbohydrate, lower-protein diet based on the USDA food guide pyramid actually reduced the effectiveness of exercise," said Dr. Layman Forty-eight adult women participated in Layman's four-month study, published in the August 2007 edition of *The Journal of Nutrition*. One group ate a protein-rich diet designed to contain specific levels of leucine; a second group consumed a diet based on the food guide pyramid, which contained higher amounts of carbohydrates. Both groups consumed the same number of calories, but the first group substituted high-quality protein foods, such as meats, dairy, eggs, and nuts, for foods high in carbohydrates, such as breads, rice, cereal, pasta, and potatoes.

"Both diets work because, when you restrict calories, you lose weight. But the people on the higher-protein diet lost more weight. Some people refer to this as the metabolic advantage of a protein-rich diet," said Layman.

The study included two levels of exercise. "For one group, we recommended that they add walking to their lives. They usually walked two to three times a week, less than one hundred minutes of added exercise," the researcher said.

The other group was required to engage in five thirty-minute walking sessions and two thirty-minute weightlifting sessions per week. In both groups of dieters, the required exercise program helped spare lean muscle tissue and target fat loss. But, in the protein-rich, high-exercise group, Layman noted a statistically significant effect. That group lost even more weight, and almost 100 percent of the weight loss was fat. In the high-carbohydrate, high-exercise group, as much as 25–30 percent of the weight lost was muscle.

"The protein-rich diet dramatically lowered triglycerides and had a statistically significant effect on trunk fat, both risk factors associated with heart disease," he said. "Exercise helped dieters lose an even greater percentage of body fat from the abdominal area."

The protein-rich diet works so well because it contains a high-level leucine. Leucine, working together with insulin, helps stimulate protein synthesis in muscle. "The diet works because the extra protein reduces muscle loss while the low-carbohydrate component gives you low insulin, allowing you to burn fat," he said.

"We believe a diet based on the food pyramid actually does not provide enough leucine for adults to maintain healthy muscles. The average American diet contains four or five grams of leucine, but to get the metabolic effects we're seeing, you need nine or ten grams," he noted.

Dr. Layman's recommendation of .73 grams of protein per pound of body weight is the ideal amount to burn fat while retaining muscle. Precisely the same findings discovered with Dr. Peter Lemon.

This is the key in balancing carbohydrates, protein, and fat. If leucine levels remain elevated, it's safe to say you're building or keeping muscle, not losing it and burning fat. I explain later what specific foods you need to consume daily to get this essential amino acid. Women need not be turned off by "muscle-building" amino acids. We are not talking big bulky muscles, but a lean and feminine physique that burns more calories per hour and can be found in specific proteins.

DOES PROTEIN EXCRETE CALCIUM?

I read recently that calcium is excreted if an individual eats 140 grams of protein per day. This claim holds no water. Special interest groups and a few nutritionists since the 1970s have been making claims that moderate- to high-protein diets make the body excrete more calcium, which could weaken bones. While others claim the opposite, recent research strongly suggests that the protein proponents were right all along. The studies show that a diet high in protein not only keeps your bones healthy, it can actually significantly slow down the bone loss that leads to osteoporosis (thin, brittle bones that break easily).

Research since 1998 in the *American Journal of Clinical Nutrition* shows that dietary protein for building and maintaining strong bones is significant on protein diets that are high to moderate. A study of a number of young women compared the effects on calcium absorption in a low-protein and a high-protein diet. The result?

Calcium absorption from food was much lower on the low-protein (RDA's recommendation) diet.

WHAT DOES THIS MEAN FOR YOU?

Males will be safe for body fat loss while retaining muscle tissue at forty grams of protein at three different settings. The three meals will each contain forty grams of protein; the other two will be either less or more depending on your desired weight. I lay this out for you in a simple way in Chapter 8.

The meals should not ever exceed fifty grams—as this will take a toll on your metabolism, liver, and kidneys. Females will be safe for body fat loss at twenty grams of protein at three different settings. The three meals will each contain twenty grams of protein; the other two will be either less or more depending on your desired weight. Again, you should never exceed twenty-five grams in a three-hour setting, regardless of your current size.

The Transform Diet recommends .73 grams of protein per pound of your target or future body weight. It sounds almost ridiculous and maybe fanatical to try to get the precise amount in each meal, right? Wrong. Like carbohydrates, you will know after a few days what to look for to get the protein to these requirements.

A diet that contains protein in each meal doesn't mean high protein, as long as you eat accordingly. As you have read, I have done the homework for you by breaking down individual meals every three hours. By simply adjusting meals three and five, you need to eat to the exact weight of where you want to be, not exceeding what I have given you. This recommendation is the safest, most effective way to burn body fat while preserving muscle tissue.

FATS

There are four basic types of fats you need to concern yourself with: saturated, monounsaturated, polyunsaturated, and trans fats. Cholesterol is a sterol. It is not a true fat, but a fatlike substance that exists in animal foods and body cells. The types of fats you need to consume on a daily basis are monounsaturated and polyunsaturated fats.

Fats, like fiber, control the entry rate of carbohydrates into the bloodstream. Good fats actually have no effect on insulin; however, they drastically control hunger and affect body fat levels. The only way you can get lean is to steer clear of trans fats (donuts, fast food, etc.) on a daily basis.

Low amounts of saturated fat can be good. In fact, I like animal fats because they don't allow the depletion of vitamin A that leads to autoimmune diseases and underactive thyroid, causing weight gain, along with so many other health problems.

The two types of fat that will transform your body are monounsaturated and polyunsaturated. It's these very fats that get you lean when eaten at the right times in the right amounts. You hear fat, you think fat. Think again.

According to health specialist Anne Collins, "Monounsaturated fat is considered to be probably the healthiest type of general fat. It has none of the adverse effects associated with saturated fats, or trans fats. The high consumption of olive oil in Mediterranean countries is considered one of the reasons why these countries have lower levels of heart disease.

She continues, "Polyunsaturated fat is healthier than saturated fats. It is also an essential element in our diet because polyunsaturated fat includes a special family of essential fatty acids (which the human body cannot manufacture for itself) called Omega-3 and Omega-6 fatty acids."

WHICH FATS ARE BEST AND HOW MUCH?

You need good fats with every meal of every day. It's one of the quickest ways to a hardened physique. A fantastic trick with the eating of good fats is, it releases a powerful hormone called CCK or Cholecystokinin from your stomach. It's the one that tells your brain you're satisfied. It can be released every time you eat. You just have to choose the right fat with each meal with the precise amount.

Remember, when it comes to the amount of fat in each meal, more is not better and less is not good either. Simply put, do not exceed 18 grams of fat per meal, and do not eat less than 6 grams per meal.

1. Flaxseed: I know of no other fat we can buy that contains monounsaturated fat, polyunsaturated fat (Omega-3), dietary fiber, and lignans so concentrated in a single tablespoon. Omega-3s are typically found in fish, but the flaxseed contains high amounts in a small dose. It's why flaxseed without question is your number one choice. There is nothing even close, and that's not even the good part.

My recommendation is two tablespoons per day. Flaxseed is a highly efficient food, it is full of lignans—a plant chemical that acts like a powerful hormone by controlling estrogen levels in men and women—and that may be its greatest characteristic.

It's this fat and fiber of the flaxseed that will be extraordinary in breaking up fatty tissue throughout your body. I don't know any substance like it. I'm not sure it's received the praise it deserves. I'm going to do it justice in Chapter 5.

Do not exceed four tablespoons per day. This powerful hormone actually has shown some side effects at higher dosages, which proves just how powerful it really is. This is the ultimate fat choice and your daily staple.

2. Almonds and walnuts: My second favorite—the almond—contains fiber, monounsaturated fat, and polyunsaturated fat, but no Omega-3s. Eat twelve almonds, (natural, raw, not salted) per meal, but not any more in a three-hour period. One almond contains seven calories and 0.59 grams of fat. The fiber in the almond will not allow insulin to spike. It's also a powerful antioxidant and a great source of magnesium—the mineral you need to produce energy and absorb potassium. The almond prevents cravings because it balances blood sugar levels. Almonds have the highest protein content of any nut and may be highly beneficial to the vegetarian or vegan.

The most interesting thing is their ability to actually block calories. Research shows the cell walls of the almond reduce the absorption of their fat. Almonds are a very powerful monounsaturated fat. You need to be sure not eat more than twelve per meal. By doing this, your physique will tighten and harden by eating the precise amount.

The walnut has 25 percent more saturated fat than the almond per serving, with many of the same benefits and does have the Omega-3 fat. I prefer the almond for taste as much as its proven ability to block calories.

3. Extra Virgin Olive Oil: The Mediterranean Diet will tell you it's number one, because of the studies they have done. However, without fiber or polyunsaturated fat, I have to disagree. Yes, polyunsaturated fat in high amounts can do more harm than good, but with my meal plan in Chapter 8, you needn't worry about that. This special oil will lower cholesterol levels in the blood. It also lowers blood pressure and blood sugar levels. With this oil, you have to be careful as it's poured out. One tablespoon has fourteen grams of monounsaturated fat. Always buy virgin or extra virgin as this means it's unrefined.

4. Avocados: Avocados, like almonds, contain oleic acid, a monounsaturated fat that helps to lower cholesterol. The perfect amount of avocado you should eat with one meal is one-quarter— that size gives you all the benefits without the storage of body fat. Avocados contain eighty-one micrograms of the carotenoid lutein, which studies suggest maintain healthy eyes. Avocados contribute nearly twenty vitamins, minerals and phytonutrients, including vitamin E, vitamin C, foliate, fiber, iron, and potassium, with nineteen micrograms of beta-carotene. Avocados act as a "nutrient booster" by enabling the body to absorb more fat-soluble nutrients, such as alpha- and beta-carotene. Not too bad for being number four on this list. The other three do a better job of external hardening of the body.

5. Peanut Butter: Other nutritionist have it in their top three, but the reason it isn't higher for me is the external effects on the human body. The internal effects are similar to olive oil. Here is the scoop: a tablespoon can have a negative effect because you hold more water than usual on the body, something that will frustrate the dieter. There are other compounds in peanut butter that create the soft look on many individuals—especially if the peanut butter is a brand name and not pure organic peanuts. Peanut butter creates a layer of water between the skin and muscle, which can be frustrating for those in search of defined abs.

I also don't like peanuts as they are the number one food allergy to humans, soy being second. Read the label. Stay away from hydrogenated anything, which is in many store-brand peanut butters. It's a killer for the midsection. Eating peanut butter doesn't make sense in the first twelve weeks or until you see serious results. After that, I would use it in moderation.

Chapter 5

━━━━◆━━━━

The Big Three

THE RAW OAT

Why the raw oat? Let's start with this. According to biochemist Dr. Barry Sears, there are only two common foods on this planet that contain Gamma Linolenic Acid (GLA). They are human breast milk and raw oats. GLA is an essential fatty acid (a good fat) in the Omega-6 family. Although there are only trace amounts found in oatmeal, it shows just how special this carbohydrate really is.

In 1997, the Food and Drug Administration actually allowed raw oats (and this is rare) to carry a label claiming it may reduce the risk of heart disease when combined with a low-fat diet. What other starch carbohydrate gets that allowance?

There are two types of fiber found in oatmeal: soluble and insoluble. Both are undigested carbohydrates—therefore they are not absorbed into the bloodstream. Instead of being used as energy, fiber is excreted from our bodies. Soluble fiber forms a gel-like substance when mixed with liquid, while insoluble fiber does not. Insoluble fiber passes through our intestines largely intact.

What does all this mean? The insoluble fiber promotes regular bowel movements and prevents constipation. It removes toxic waste through the colon in less time as it controls the pH (acidity) in the intestines—preventing colon cancer by keeping an optimal pH in the intestines to prevent microbes from producing cancerous substances.

The soluble fiber binds with fatty acids, prolonging stomach-emptying time so that sugar is released and absorbed more slowly. Did you catch that? Fiber acts like a brake on the rate of entry for the absorption of other carbohydrates into the bloodstream.

Soluble fiber also significantly lowers total cholesterol and the LDL (bad cholesterol), reducing the risk of heart disease. The fiber also regulates blood sugar for people with diabetes. It's like oatmeal has a mind of its own. Slow-cooked is best; however, how realistic is it for the working population to spend time preparing a bowl of oatmeal? Maybe on the weekends. In the Transform Diet, raw oatmeal will be the staple in your blender every morning.

What makes the oat so special?

Gluten is the protein part of wheat, rye, barley, and other related grains. However, gluten is not found in oats. It's yet another reason why this grain is so amazing. Some people cannot tolerate gluten when it comes in contact with the small intestine. The condition is known as celiac disease.

Gluten injures the lining of the small intestine resulting in bloating, gas, abdominal cramps, and diarrhea. If patients can eliminate gluten completely from the diet, the lining of the intestine has an opportunity to heal itself.

The oat is a grain that deserves the highest praise, as it is believed safe in patients with celiac disease—although where it's made can change everything. The problem with oat products is not the grain, but the manufacturing process. When oats are processed in the same facilities as wheat, contamination can occur—even with the best cleaning protocol. However, most celiac patients can tolerate pure oat products.

The January 9, 2008, issue of *ScienceDaily* states, "A new scientific review of the most current research shows the link between eating oatmeal and cholesterol reduction to be stronger than when the FDA initially approved the health claim's appearance on food labels in 1997." Here is what they found out about benefits of eating oatmeal:

- Reduces the risk for elevated blood pressure Type 2 diabetes and weight gain
- Reduces LDL cholesterol during weight loss
- Provides favorable changes in the physical characteristics of LDL cholesterol particles, making them less susceptible to oxidation (oxidation is thought to lead to hardening of the arteries.)
- Supplies unique compounds that may lead to reducing early hardening of the arteries
- Total cholesterol levels are lowered through oat consumption
- LDL (the "bad" cholesterol) is reduced without adverse effects on HDL cholesterol (the "good" cholesterol), or triglyceride concentrations.

Dr. James W. Anderson, professor of medicine and clinical nutrition at the University of Kentucky College of Medicine, says "Since the eighties, oatmeal has been scientifically recognized for its heart health benefits, and the latest research shows this evidence endures the test of time and should be embraced as a lifestyle option for the millions of Americans at-risk for heart disease."

HOW MUCH ENERGY DOES THE RAW OAT PROVIDE?

My good friend, Keith Reilly, found out just how powerful the oat is. He was in charge of taking an LDS youth group of mostly Eagle Scouts to the Sierra Mountains. The climb that reached nearly nine thousand feet was all this thirty-five-year-old male could handle. With a fifty-five-pound backpack, and no experience in this field, he arrived last at the top of the treacherous climb, nearly two days later. Exhausted and unable to move, the Eagle Scouts ridiculed and harassed him about how old and tired he was. Twenty-four hours later, they had to leave the site and head back down the mountain; everyone considered it a very tough situation.

Dreading the walk back and unable to leave anything behind, Reilly was forced to carry the same amount of weight as when he came up. The only item in his backpack he could dispose of was twelve packs of oatmeal. So, he mixed it in water and drank it raw. Not thinking anything of it, he began his journey back down the hill. He felt sick to his stomach and wondered why he had eaten all of that oatmeal because it was still the same weight—regardless of whether it was in his stomach or backpack. What he didn't realize was that his backpack would not allow the oats to be broken down like they did in his pancreas. The oatmeal entered his bloodstream like a high-octane racing fuel in a Formula One car. Because of its low glycemic index, oatmeal yields sustained energy as it is released slowly, and it also does not spike insulin levels. Oatmeal has been proven to prolong energy throughout the course of an entire day. Eight hours later and to the amazement of everyone, he was jogging the last half mile. In fact, he was laughing at everyone, as he sprinted out to the parking lot where his car was parked. As the Eagle Scouts finished one by one, they were in shock to see he had finished first. Keith, who is not even a coffee drinker, couldn't believe what the oats had done to his body.

Marathon runners and triathletes have known about this information for years, but most have not revealed this coveted trick. Of course, many of the top athletes want to keep their secret, as it's a big advantage if their opponents don't know or think to use these carbohydrates. Instead, many claim they still eat pasta before a run.

The raw oat is the key to hardening your body. When eaten daily, it's the premier complex carbohydrate protein blend, as it will aid in energy, strength, recovery, and overall wellbeing.

Flaxseed

The Washington Post reported that Olympic gold-medalist Marion Jones had acknowledged in a letter to close family and friends that while preparing for the 2000 Olympics it was flaxseed oil—not performance-enhancing drugs—that helped her win four gold medals. Like Jones, Major League Baseball superstar Barry Bonds has denied knowingly doing anything wrong by stating that it was flaxseed that helped him hit more than seventy home runs. So let's understand this: both athletes could have chosen any substance in the Universe and yet they both claimed that using flaxseed was the essential role and key ingredient to putting their careers over the top? Although the claims were unsubstantiated, the hype is not.

What makes the flaxseed so powerful? Flaxseeds contain high levels of lignans, a natural antioxidant and a member of the family of plant estrogens (phytoestrogens). Many plant foods contain lignans; however, flaxseed has at least seventy-five times more than any other food. Its closest competitors (wheat bran, buckwheat, rye, millet, oats, and soybeans) are not even close. To get the lignans that are in just two tablespoons of flaxseed, you would need to eat thirty cups of raw broccoli.

Dr. Ann Louise Gittleman, PhD says, "Ground-up flaxseeds are also the highest source of lignans, an estrogen modulating substance that is very protective against estrogen dependent cancers—from breast cancer to prostate cancer—so you get a double whammy when you use ground-up flax. And, it contains 50 percent soluble fibers and 50 percent insoluble fibers, so you get the regulating effects of the fiber as well as the effects of blood sugar stabilization, and even cholesterol regulation. So I am the biggest believer in ground-up flax."

PSYLLIUM VS. FLAXSEED

Gittleman says, "Psyllium can become gooey; it absorbs lots of water in the system, so people's bowels can become quite dehydrated. Overuse of psyllium can actually strip the bowel of beneficial bacterium."

In a 1997 double-blind study, Dr. Tarpila S. Kivinen, from the Department of Pharmacology at the University of Tampere, studied fifty-five people with chronic constipation caused by Irritable Bowel Syndrome. The study subjects received either ground flaxseed or psyllium seed (a well-known treatment for constipation) daily for three months. Those taking flaxseed had significantly fewer problems with constipation, abdominal pain, and bloating than those taking psyllium. The flaxseed group had even further improvements in constipation and bloating while continuing their treatment in the three months after the double-blind study ended. The researcher concluded that flaxseed relieved constipation more effectively than psyllium.

THE BENEFITS OF FLAXSEED

Health experts Jose Antonio of the International Society of Sports Nutrition, Roger Clemens of the University of Southern California, Lisa Hark of the University of Pennsylvania School of Medicine, and Hector Lopez of Physicians Pioneering Performance collaborated and found that Omega-3s in flaxseed decrease the amount of fat in our bloodstream and help reduce the risk of a heart attack. Omega-3s are also believed to strengthen muscles and bones—and they may keep tissues elastic so that blood vessels can maintain a lower blood pressure and the heart doesn't need to pump as hard.

Flaxseed, as they point out, also helps an athlete to recover from injuries. The Omega-3s affect the production of cytokines, which are involved in regulating inflammation associated with joint pain, stiffness, and swelling. They also increase the body's sensitivity to the effects of insulin, which allows fatigued muscles to absorb more glucose, amino acids, and other nutrients needed for repair. Omega-3 fatty acids in particular have been shown to help lower cholesterol, as well as improve overall heart health. But since we can't make them, we have to eat substances that contain these omegas.

Wendy Demark-Wahnefried, an associate research professor and nutrition researcher in the department of surgery at Duke University, states that the "flaxseed is the richest source of plant-based Omega-3 fatty acids, which have been shown to reduce tumor growth in animals. In addition, flaxseed has a high lignan content—very complex, fiber-related compounds that bind testosterone in the gastrointestinal tract—and may play a role in suppressing the growth of prostate cancer cells."

The lignans found in flaxseed act like hormones in the body. Lignans actually bind the existing hormones in the body, bringing your hormones into the optimal balance. The great news is that phytoestrogens cannot be converted to estrogen. Studies have shown that four tablespoons of flaxseed per day can act like a daily dose of Novaldex or Tamoxifen (powerful prescription anti-estrogen pills) without the side effects.

It appears that lignans block the enzyme necessary for converting testosterone to estrogen. When the enzyme is blocked, testosterone is spared because it is not being converted to estrogen. In what you could visualize as a seesaw-like action, the ratio of testosterone to estrogen begins to move back in favor of testosterone—resulting in a better sex life, more energy, and lower body fat.

The action of lignans in sparing testosterone may hold greater implications than the obvious. Lack or loss of sexual desire in men and women is oftentimes associated with low testosterone levels. By preserving testosterone, many men and women may be able to retain or regain their sexual vigor. In fact, agents that block the conversion of testosterone to estrogen have been shown to increase testosterone levels by as much as 10 percent.

The ratio of testosterone to estrogen moves back in favor of testosterone to make the forty-year-old adult male feel like a twenty-year-old kid again. Lignans can also help in preventing "man breast-syndrome." It's the syndrome where too much testosterone in the body spills over into estrogen given the man a feminine, soft, big-chested look.

FLAXSEED EFFECTS ON WOMEN

Doctors Marian Verbruggen, PhD in food chemistry from the Wageningen University in the Netherlands, and Jocelyn Mathern, a nutrition and corporate fitness expert from North Dakota State University, studied the lignans found in flaxseed, and here is what they found:

"Men and women have hormones in their bodies, e.g., testosterone, estrogen, and progesterone. The amount of hormones circulating in our bodies varies throughout our life. They influence our health and how we feel. Lignans have a structure that is similar to that of human estrogen. That is why they also are called phytoestrogens (plant estrogens) that can help balance hormone levels in the body."

The anti-estrogenic activity of flaxseed-derived lignans may reduce breast carcinogenesis and metastasis (the ability of cancer cells to migrate to other parts of the body). Women who have breast cancer generally have a 10–20 percent higher concentration of the estrogen hormone estradiol. The anti-estrogen activity allows it to be pushed out of the body. In doing so, it balances the correct ratio of estrogen to testosterone in women.

What do you think happens when a woman has too much estrogen? She typically has increased body fat, moodiness, lack of energy, and decreased sex drive. By balancing the hormones with lignans, she now increases her energy, which changes her physically, mentally, and emotionally.

According to a French study published in the March 21, 2007, issue *Journal of the National Cancer Institute*, "A diet rich in estrogen-like compounds found in flaxseed may help curb breast cancer after menopause." The study included about 58,000 postmenopausal French women who were followed for an average of more than seven years.

SIDE EFFECTS OF FLAXSEED

Too much flaxseed may have some side effects that need to be mentioned. The lignans contain a substance known as cyanogenic glycosides. Foods such as yams and lima beans also carry these substances. Cyanogenic glycosides metabolize into another substance known as SCN or thiocyanate. This is a chemical that has the potential to suppress the thyroid's ability to metabolize iodine, which can lead to goiter (enlargement of the thyroid gland). These studies were done at high dosages over eighteen months. I recommend not exceeding four tablespoons per day, but not less than two either. Remember, vitamin A and its many positive benefits can be toxic at high dosages. The same is true with flaxseed.

Unground flaxseed is not digestible and, as a result, it will not supply the body with the necessary lignans or ALA. For optimum nutrient value, use ground flaxseeds instead of flax oil. Flax oil contains Omega-3 fatty acids, but it does *not* contain the beneficial lignans and fiber. The lignan and fiber are removed in the production process.

FLAXSEED'S EFFECT ON PEOPLE

- Flax contains a special fiber called mucilage. Mucilage helps stabilize blood sugar levels, and is a natural laxative.

- Ground flaxseed is rich in protein, B vitamins, vitamin E, beta-carotene, calcium, potassium, magnesium, manganese, and zinc.

- Women report relief from minor symptoms such as hot flashes, anxiety, and irritability.

- The lignans found in flaxseed are said to have anti-tumor effects.

- The lubricative properties of flaxseed are believed to help reduce symptoms of arthritis.

- Four tablespoons of flaxseed provides 240 milligrams of potassium and 120 milligrams of calcium (a medium-sized banana has 450 milligrams of potassium).

- Flax decreases inflammation. Inflammation causes migraines, lupus, MS, psoriasis, and rheumatoid arthritis. Flax is also helpful to people suffering with Crohn's disease and celiac.

- Two tablespoons of flaxseed has 2,400 milligrams of Alpha-linolenic acid (Omega-3, not to be confused with the fish version of Omega-3s). Walnuts and canola oil are the next highest and they have only about 10 percent in comparison.

- Charlemagne the Great considered flax so healthy that he passed laws requiring its consumption.

- According to the American Academy of Dermatology, the lignans found in flaxseed can help men and women with hair loss and the thinning of hair. It has been proven that flaxseed plays a role in this.

Flaxseed breakdown:

Supplement Facts

Serving Size 2 Tbsp (15 g)
Servings Per Container 30

Amount Per Serving

Calories 90   Calories from Fat 60

	% Daily Value*
Total Fat 7 g	**11%**
Saturated Fat 0 g	**0%**
Polyunsaturated Fat 4 g	
Monounsaturated Fat 1 g	
Cholesterol 0 mg	**0%**
Sodium 0 mg	**0%**
Total Carbohydrate 5 g	**2%**
Dietary Fiber 3 g	**12%**
Insoluble Fiber 2 g	
Soluble Fiber 1 g	

Trace Vitamins

Vitamin C 75 mcg	**0%**
Vitamin B-1 (Thiamin) 79 mcg	**5%**
Vitamin B-2 (Riboflavin) 34 mcg	**2%**
Vitamin B-6 (Pyridoxine Hcl) 90 mcg	**7%**
Niacin 480 mcg	**2%**
Pantothenic Acid 85 mcg	**2%**
Folic Acid 16 mcg	**4%**

Tocopherols (Vit-E)

Alpha-Tocopherol 8 mcg	†
Delta-Tocopherol 6 mcg	†
Gamma-Tocopherol 4 mcg	†

Trace Minerals

Calcium 30 mg	**3%**
Copper 150 mcg	**7%**
Iron 750 mcg	**4%**
Magnesium 60 mcg	**15%**
Manganese 30 mcg	**0%**
Phosphorus 93 mg	**6%**
Potassium 120 mg	**3%**
Zinc 750 mcg	**2%**

Amino Acids (Protein) 2645 mg   **6%**

Alanine 125 mg	†
Arginine 270 mg	†
Aspartic Acid 270 mg	†
Cystine 30 mg	†
Glutamic Acid 580 mg	†
Glycine 170 mg	†
Histidine 60 mg	†
Isoleucine 115 mg	†
Leucine 170 mg	†
Lysine 115 mg	†
Methionine 40 mg	†
Phenylalanine 130 mg	†
Proline 100 mg	†
Serine 130 mg	†
Threonine 100 mg	†
Tryptophan 50 mg	†
Tyrosine 60 mg	†
Valine 130 mg	†

Essential Fatty Acids

Omega-3 (alpha-linolenic acid) 3000 mg	†
Omega-6 (linolenic acid) 1000 mg	†

Monounsaturated Fatty Acids

Omega-9 1000 mg	†

Phyto-Nutrients

Lignans (SDG) 110-300 mg	†
Phenolic Acids 100 mg	†
Flavonoids 5 mg	†
Phytic Acid 320 mg	†

* Percent Daily Values (DV) are based on a 2,000 calorie diet.
† Daily Value not established.

WHEY PROTEIN

Whey protein, a byproduct of cheese, is manufactured from cow's milk. Milk contains two major types of protein: casein and whey. Whey wasn't acknowledged until about twenty-five years ago. It was traditionally thought to be worthless until someone decided to examine this "waste" product. What seemed to be typical dairy product on the surface was far from it when broken down and metabolized in the body. It was discovered that whey was loaded with a highly bioactive protein that is more similar to the protein found in human breast milk than any other known source. These proteins dissolved well in water, were highly digestible, and contained an even better amino acid profile than the highly regarded egg.

For years, protein powders have tasted like chalky, thick, nasty stuff with floaters in it. I suppose twenty years ago when soy protein powders came on the market, they spoiled it for anyone who dared to try. To everyone's surprise, in the past three years, whey protein has changed all that. In fact, when you look at protein powder now, it has the consistency of chocolate milk or the thickness of a milkshake—depending on how much liquid you choose to add.

Depending on the brand, some even taste like Nestle Quik or Ovaltine. When you add ice to these powders and mix in water, they now start to taste like a smoothie from Smoothie King—they are delicious. As powders continue to grow in revenue, so does the quality and taste. You no longer need a blender to make a protein shake. If you have a spoon and a cup with water, believe it or not, you have something that is healthy and tastes better than good.

A recent article on Buzzle.com said this about whey protein, "Scientists have come a long way in their development of protein supplements, including how they taste. Even recently, the best you could hope for with a protein shake was that you could choke it down in spite of its chalky taste and consistency. Now they actually taste good. Today, there are plenty of protein powders and meal replacement shakes on the market.

"The key is finding the best quality products with the highest level of bioavailability. Avoid soy proteins, as these are the cheapest products you can buy and typically are genetically modified. Genetic modification means scientists have altered the organism from its natural state, a practice discouraged by most non-soy-paid scientists. Do your own independent research if you like, but always consider the source. Take with a grain of salt the comments of 'specialists' who are paid by companies to say theirs is the best stuff for your body."

So just how good is whey protein for both men and women? There is a rating system for proteins called the BV rating or Biological Value rating system. The rating measures the amount of protein (nitrogen) absorbed in the human body. The more protein absorbed and used by the body, the higher the Biological Value.

The whole egg set the standard for the biological value rating system in 1911. The egg was considered the greatest BV-rated protein you could eat—due to 100 percent of its protein being absorbed. So, the egg earned a BV rating of 100. Nearly twenty-five years ago when whey protein was eventually measured using the biological value rating system, it received a BV rating of 104. It left everyone baffled and the rating system needed to be revamped. For now, 100 is not really 100, it's a 104.

What does this mean? It means that whey was literally off the charts for human absorption. It also meant that critics questioned whey's quick absorption rate. Does it leave our body too quickly and drop the blood sugar levels, which would then store excess body fat? Good question, but here is the catch: fiber is the key to slowing down absorption and keeping insulin levels from spiking—by adding raw oats with flaxseed to whey protein, they create arguably the greatest concoction of a meal we can feed ourselves.

The problem with raw whey is that it contains too much undesirable lactose, fat, and cholesterol. A few years ago, two new, major processes were developed, that have the ability to extract the proteins from whey while preserving their integrity. These processes are micro-filtration (where the proteins are physically separated by a microscopic filter) and ion exchange (where proteins are extracted by taking advantage of their specific electronic charges). Both of these processes yield a high-quality, low-lactose, low-fat whey protein. In fact, pure iso whey protein powders are a little more expensive, but all lactose and fat have been removed in the filtration process, making it a prime choice for lactose-intolerant people.

BENEFITS OF WHEY PROTEIN

Jennifer Warner's July 2005 article on WebMD Health News shows adding whey to a high-carbohydrate meal may help people with diabetes keep their blood sugar levels under control. Researchers found drinking a whey supplement mixed with water along with a meal, like mashed potatoes with meatballs, prevented the dramatic spikes in blood sugar levels. Researchers say the results suggest that whey aids in blood sugar regulation by stimulating the production of the hormone insulin in the pancreas. The study showed that rises in blood sugar levels after lunch were reduced by 21 percent with whey supplementation. The findings suggest that whey proteins may attenuate blood sugar surges throughout the day.

OTHER FINDINGS

- A European research group also reported that whey protein lowers cortisol levels. Cortisol is a hormone released by your adrenal glands in response to either physical or emotional stress. High levels of cortisol will lead to protein breakdown.

- In one trial carried in the *Journal of Applied Physiology*, Canadian scientists found that after three months of supplementation, whey protein was more effective at improving exercise performance than casein. The whey protein group also lost body fat and reported feeling far more energetic.

- Scientists from Australia have reported that a whey protein isolate is far superior to casein for muscle growth. Thirteen subjects were given either whey isolate or casein while they took part in a weight-training program for ten weeks. Results showed that the 100 percent whey isolate was more effective at increasing muscle mass. Test subjects using whey gained more than ten pounds of muscle, while those using casein gained only two pounds. Those using whey also gained more strength, although both proteins seemed to prevent the typical drop in plasma glutamine levels that occurs with exercise.

- A recent study in Europe compared whey protein to casein, the primary protein in milk. They found that older men who consumed whey protein showed greater protein synthesis, or growth, which helped limit muscle loss over time than with casein.

ACCORDING TO THE WHEY PROTEIN INSTITUTE:

- Whey protein is a naturally complete protein—meaning it contains all of the essential amino acids (building blocks of protein) that help you lose body fat and overall body composition.
- Whey protein contains the highest levels of branched chained amino acids of any other food we can eat.
- The amino acid leucine—found in whey protein—has approximately 50 percent more found than in soy protein.
- Recent studies by Dr. Donald Layman, a professor at the University of Illinois, found that leucine is the central key amino to preserve lean muscle tissue while promoting fat loss.
- Whey protein helps to stabilize blood glucose levels by slowing the absorption of glucose into the bloodstream. This, in turn, reduces hunger by lowering insulin levels and making it easier for the body to burn fat.
- Whey has two appetite suppressing hormones: CCK (cholecystokinin) and GLP-1 (glucagon-like peptide 1). These help to control food intake considerably at the next meal.
- At the 2003 annual meeting of the American Cancer Society, research showed high levels of cysteine had nearly a 60 percent reduction in the risk of breast cancer compared to lower levels of cysteine. Studies have shown that whey protein, rich in the amino acid cysteine, provides an extra boost to the immune system by raising glutathione levels. This has been shown to

reduce the risk of infection and improve the responsiveness of the immune system.

- Whey protein helps stop the onset of Type 2 diabetes. It helps the blood glucose levels to remain normal.

- Whey is now a key ingredient of infant formulas—including those for premature infants. Certain types of whey formulas have been shown to reduce crying in colicky infants. When breastfeeding is not an option, whey is considered the next-best choice. Breast milk is found to have the same components as whey protein.

- Whey protein is now the superior choice for expectant mothers according to doctors.

- Whey proteins do more than build muscle and repair tissue—they create antibodies, which are part of the enzyme and hormonal systems, which neutralize foreign objects, such as bacteria and viruses.

- Whey protein helps athletes maintain a healthy immune system by increasing the levels of glutathione in the body. Glutathione is an anti-oxidant required for a healthy immune system, and exercise and resistance training may reduce glutathione levels. Whey protein helps keep athletes healthy and strong to perform their best.

- Whey protein has been shown through animal and in vitro studies to inhibit the growth of several types of cancer tumors. Dr. Thomas Badger, head of the Arkansas Children's Nutrition Center in Little Rock, found that feeding rats whey protein resulted in their developing 50 percent fewer tumors than rats fed casein. The rats fed whey protein also developed fewer tumors than rats fed soy protein and the tumors took longer to develop.

- Whey protein is a very high quality protein and is often the preferred choice for high protein products recommended by physicians following surgery or burn therapy.

- Whey protein also contains components with protective anti-microbial properties, such as lactoferrin. In recent years, companies have introduced mouthwashes and oral care products containing these protective whey protein components.

Chapter 6

Water Intake

On April 3, 2008, Dr. Stanley Goldfarb, a nephrologist at the hospital of the University of Pennsylvania, dropped a bombshell, "If you're thirsty, drink," says Goldfarb. "If you're not thirsty, you needn't drink. Drinking eight glasses of water per day is a myth."

Goldfarb continued, "Water helping you excrete toxins was not verified by any scientific study since kidneys do the job regardless of how much water you consume." Adding a few extra glasses of water each day has limited effect. "It's such a tiny part of what's in the body. It's very unlikely that one's getting any benefit. As for upping your intake to improve skin tone or reduce headaches: There was never a scientific basis for it," Goldfarb said.

Goldfarb's conclusion—if you are an athlete, have certain diseases, or live in hot, dry climates, you might need to increase your fluid intake. Otherwise, more water does not translate to better health and apparently is lacking in any scientific basis.

The CBS News anchor Katie Couric who first reported the story said, "The researchers looked at all of the studies out there and found no evidence that drinking lots of water has lots of benefits." CBS News also said, "No significant studies have ever been done."

I strongly disagree with Dr. Stanley Goldfarb's theories. Numerous studies have been done that support the benefits of drinking water.

STUDIES THAT SUPPORT WATER INTAKE

"Drinking Water Can Help Your Diet": *ScienceDaily* **(Feb. 5, 2003)**—Drinking water can help you in your efforts to lose weight, says a Wake Forest University Baptist Medical Center nutritionist. "Water can decrease your appetite," said Mara Z. Vitolins, R.D., Dr. P.H., assistant professor of public health sciences (epidemiology). "It is hard to distinguish between being thirsty and being hungry, so try drinking water and waiting twenty to thirty minutes to see if you're still hungry." Vitolins, who also is part of the Center for Research on Human Nutrition and Chronic Disease Prevention, added that drinking water also may help you cut calories.

"Water is an important nutrient and is vital for a variety of bodily functions and processes, including removal of waste products, carrying nutrients, and regulating body temperature. Water helps reduce fluid retention, and helps keep bowel functions normal. I think many people would greatly benefit by recording the amount of water they drink in a day," Vitolins said. "Many folks I have asked to do this are surprised at how little they drink. It is an essential nutrient, yet so few actually get enough."

In February 2004, Dr. Stella L. Volpe, PhD, R.D., and Miriam Stril, a term-endowed chair in nutrition from the University of Pennsylvania, looked very seriously at how much fluid the body really needs. Both are members of the Institute of Medicine's National Academics of Sciences.

These doctors published the first ever "Dietary Reference Intakes" for water and electrolytes such as sodium and potassium chloride (which control the movement of water in and out of the cells of your muscle and organs), telling us their water-intake recommendations.

The Institute of Medicine specialists spent two years examining hundreds of studies from peer-reviewed scientific journals on everything from normal fluid balance and kidney function, to fluid needs for those who are ill.

The panel concluded that "healthy, sedentary, ages nineteen to fifty men who live in temperate climate are adequately hydrated when they get 3.7 liters or one gallon of water, and 2.7 liters or 91 ounces of water for women." Again, these are people who don't exercise, and are considered couch potatoes.

In the December 2004 issue of *The Journal of Clinical Endocrinology and Metabolism,* researchers in Germany reported that water consumption increases the rate at which people burn calories.

Michael Boschmann, MD, and colleagues from Berlin's Franz-Volhard Clinical Research Center tracked energy expenditures among seven men and seven women who were healthy and not overweight. After drinking approximately seventeen ounces of water, the subjects' metabolic rates—or the rate at which calories are burned—increased by 30 percent for both men and women. The increases occurred within ten minutes of water consumption and reached a maximum after about thirty to forty minutes.

The study also showed that the increase in metabolic rate differed in men and women. In men, burning more fat fueled the increase in metabolism, whereas in women, an increased breakdown of carbohydrates caused the increase in metabolism.

The researchers estimate that over the course of a year, a person who increases his water consumption by 1.5 liters a day would burn an extra 17,400 calories, for a weight loss of approximately five pounds.

Dr. Donald S. Robertson graduated from Princeton University and Cornell University Medical College and achieved a master's degree in gastroenterology and nutritional sciences from the University of Colorado. Additionally, he studied at the Center for Nutritional Research at Harvard's Deaconess Hospital. He said, "The kidneys cannot function without enough water. When they do not work to capacity, some of their load is dumped to the liver. One of the liver's primary functions is to metabolize stored fat into usable energy for the body. But if the liver has to do some of the kidney's work, it cannot work at full throttle."

Dr. Anne Louis Gittleman said, "It's ironic, but consuming too little water can cause your body to retain water. Your kidneys must have adequate water to flush waste from your body. When your fluid intake is low, the kidneys hoard water."

Chair of the Wellness Institute at the Cleveland Clinic, Dr. Michael Rozen said, "It's important to drink eight glasses of water every day. It helps to move the poop and gives you better hydration. It actually cuts down on wrinkles too, because you hydrate your skin when you take it internally."

"Water: The Unexpected Blood Pressure Drug" *ScienceDaily (Feb. 8, 2000)*—"Patients who suffer from autonomic nervous system failure can turn to a new treatment for their blood pressure abnormalities: a large glass of water. Investigators at Vanderbilt's Autonomic Dysfunction Center report in the February 8 issue of the journal *Circulation* said that water has a powerful blood pressure raising effect in these patients. Water also raises blood pressure in older normal subjects, but not in young normal subjects. The studies suggest that water is an important unrecognized factor in clinical studies of blood pressure medications."

THE CHEMISTRY OF WATER

Water is the transport medium. Our bodies are approximately 70 percent water, depending on how much body fat you have. Women have less water, close to 55–60 percent. Water plays an essential role in every process in our bodies. Water is the medium for transporting nutrients to the cells and waste material from the cells. It carries brain messages and nerve impulses throughout the body. The quality of the water we drink has a major effect on the quality of our lives as I'm about to prove.

Dr. Mu Shik Jhon was one of the world's leading authorities on the structure of water. He studied at the University of Utah where he earned a PhD in chemistry in 1966.

His first book, *Significant Liquid Structures*, was co-authored with the world-famous scientist Dr. Henry Eyring. The University of Utah's chemistry building on campus is named in his honor. In 1986, Dr. Jhon presented the *Molecular Water Environment Theory* at a symposium on cancer. After nearly forty years of research on water, here are those facts:

Clean snow or pure rainwater are in this hexagonal form also known as distilled. They are considered to be the "biological form." Scientists have found that infants are born with six-sided water molecule or hexagonal clusters. The natural water found in vegetable tissue is also six-sided. The six-sided form is consistent with the fluids in our body. They considered this a perfect form of water. The question is where can we get a perfect six-sided water cluster?

- According to the experts, the six-sided hexagonal form of water allows more effective transportation of oxygen and nutrients by the blood to the cells and more effective push of inorganic material and waste elimination.

- The six-sided hexagonal water molecule improves the leaching out of toxic minerals from the body. Five-sided clusters cannot. Chemical and electrical communications between cells are best with six sides.

- Water can also configure itself into the not so good five-sided or pentagonal forms. This side is not in harmony with the fluids of the body and contributes to many illnesses and diseases.

- Biologists and chemists have found that high concentrations of five-sided water clusters are common in people with deficient immune systems.

DISTILLED WATER: THE PERFECT SIX-SIDED CLUSTER

Recent studies have allowed our world's greatest thinkers to re-examine water. They have come to one conclusion. Despite the purity of reverse osmosis, the molecular structure is a five-sided pentagonal form. It's still not suited to push waste out of the body like distilled water's six-sided cluster.

Biochemist Steve Chemiske said, "When clustered water is consumed, high frequency information is transmitted to proteins, and this wave of information is carried throughout the body like a 'wake-up call' to restore normal function."

There is still another molecular water cluster known as "random structure." This is the type that is commonly found in tap, well, and city water. This random type is the least desirable to drink since cellular detoxification is nonexistent. Also, it usually has unusable forms of minerals dissolved in it and an acid pH, which do more harm than good on the body.

Four hundred years ago, when the earth was clean, the water we drank was distilled by the sun during evaporation. Then it condensed in the atmosphere and fell back to earth as pure rain. Now the atmosphere is polluted with acidic gases from oil and byproducts. These gases add contaminants to the evaporated water, acidifying it, dissolving toxic chemicals and minerals into it, and causing mutation in its structure as it makes its way back to the earth. The rainwater of years past was not what it is today.

According to scientists, your only option to remove inorganic material and impurities is by cleansing the urea and ketones with distilled water. Distillation kills bacteria and viruses and removes complex chemicals, including pesticides, chlorine, and fluorides—and in some cases the tapeworm.

THE CAR BATTERY

Look, for instance, at the car battery and the type of water it requires. Here are two actual questions asked on a car battery web site.

Question: "Do I need to add acid to my battery?"

Answer: "No! Add distilled water only. When electrolytes are lost under normal use, the water evaporates while the acid remains in the battery. Adding acid will, therefore, alter the chemical composition of the electrolyte and cause the battery to fail more quickly. The only time electrolytes should be added is after accidental spillage. We recommend adding nothing but distilled water. No other additives have been proven to extend battery life and will decrease it."

Question: "Can I use tap, mineral, or spring water?"

Answer: "Tap water contains chemicals that are harmful to your battery as well as the others you mentioned. Even if there are just trace minerals, over four or five years of battery life, these contaminants can add up. One of the worst is water that has been softened by commonly used water softeners. Water softeners leave chlorides in the water and they are very bad for batteries. You will lose about one-third to one-half of the battery life simply by adding tap, spring, or mineral water. Use only distilled water."

So, let's get this straight. A car battery that you bought at the store has electrolytes as does the human body. Those electrolytes will be destroyed because of the chemicals added in tap, spring, or mineral water cause the battery to fail more quickly?

We are willing to not jeopardize the car battery with tap or spring water and only add distilled because the experts tell us it's the "only water" we can put into our car battery? Yet every day, we continue to drink bottled spring or tap water? How much sense does that really make? If the car battery can only used distilled, what do you think our liver, kidneys, and every other cell and organ in the body need?

The main contaminants most commonly found in our water supplies are microorganisms, heavy metals, organic chemicals, inorganic chemicals, and radioactive minerals. The most hazardous are the microorganisms: bacteria, cysts, viruses, and spores. Most city water comes from reservoirs and rivers, with the almost certainty that rainwater has washed pollutants into it. In addition to this, chemicals such as chlorine, alum, fluorine, lime, phosphates, and sodium aluminates are added to "purify" the water by killing the microorganisms.

THE TEN TYPES OF WATER

1. **Raw Water:** Raw water has millions of viruses and bacteria within its compounds. It may be as hard as limewater, or as soft as rainwater. The Environmental Protection Agency tells us that the chemicals being dumped into our rivers may be causing cancer. But, we knew that already. Raw water is a five-sided molecule.

2. **Rainwater:** Rainwater that has been distilled by the heat and sun contain no germs or bacteria. However, when falling from a cloud as rain, the chemicals, smoke, dust, and bacteria change its compounds. When rainwater reaches earth, it's not drinkable. Rainwater is a six-sided molecule.

3. **Hard Water:** Hard water has an excessive lime salt, which includes sulfates of calcium, magnesium, and carbonates—including nitrates, bacteria, viruses, silicon, copper, and sodium. The longer it filters through the soil; the more harmful it becomes to drink. Hard water is a five-sided molecule.

4. **Soft Water:** Waters taken from mountain reservoirs or lakes are considered "soft." Typically, water softeners still have inorganic materials and some bacteria. Soft water is a five-sided molecule.

5. **Snow:** Snow is frozen rain. Freezing doesn't rid water compounds from bacteria. Have you ever eaten snow? How was it? Exactly. Snow looks clean, because it's white; however, the same reasons not to use rainwater for drinking water apply. Snow is a six-sided molecule that is undrinkable.

6. **Boiled Water:** Boiling water for twenty minutes removes bacteria, but doesn't remove inorganic material. Boiled water is a five-sided molecule.

7. **Filtered Water:** Filtered water is water passed through a mechanical barrier of some type—usually a fine strainer or activated carbon. People believe filtering now purifies, but that is false. It does remove many chemicals; however, bacteria and viruses that pass through the fine mesh are a breeding ground for more problems. Remember, it's just a filter, and filters get dirty and carry bacteria. Filtered water is a five-sided molecule.

8. **Reverse Osmosis:** The process of reverse osmosis helps, but over time the equipment being used can be a breeding ground as well. It's close, but no cigar. This is a system of water purification, which allows pre-filtered water to be forced through a semi-permeable membrane to separate impurities from our drinking water. However, this membrane allows only certain molecules to pass through, providing the water pressure is exactly constant. The matter of water pressure is a problem still to be solved. Furthermore, the membrane also allows some iron and nitrate molecules to pass through. Another problem that needs to be solved. Reverse Osmosis is a five-sided molecule.

9. **De-ionized water:** Similar to distilled, but the resin beds where the de-ionizing process occurs become contaminated. The bottled water industry doesn't want to tell you that. De-ionized water is a five-sided molecule.

10. **Distilled Water:** According to the experts, distilled water is the only six-sided molecule or cluster we should drink, and the only true pure form of water—through the process of vapor elimination—is distilled. Impurities are gone. Rising vapor cannot carry dissolved solids. It will not carry disease or germs in any form. It is through the process of condensation that the final product becomes the only pure water on the planet.

Bottled water found not pure: *ScienceDaily* **(Mar. 22, 2000)—CLEVELAND—**People who buy bottled water for its perceived purity may not be getting what they're paying for: Case Western Reserve University and Ohio State University. "One of the reasons people choose to drink bottled water instead of tap water is because of the perceived purity of bottled water," the researchers observe, and indeed, thirty-nine samples of bottled water were found to be purer than the tap water. However, fifteen samples of bottled water had significantly higher bacteria levels than the tap water. Of these fifteen, the bacteria counts were more than twice as high as the most contaminated tap water sample and almost two thousand times higher than the purest tap water sample. Technicians at the Ohio Department of Health Laboratories in Columbus tested the water samples, which the researchers coded by number to eliminate the potential for bias.

The Giants (Pepsi and Coca Cola) use tap water: By CNN's Katy Byron

July 27, 2007

NEW YORK (CNN)—Pepsi-Cola announced Friday that the labels of its Aquafina brand bottled water will be changed to make it clear the product is tap water.

The new bottles will say, "The Aquafina in this bottle is purified water that originates from a public water source," or something similar, Pepsi-Cola North America spokeswoman Nicole Bradley told CNN.

The bottles are currently labeled: "Bottled at the source P.W.S." Americans spent about $2.17 billion on Aquafina last year, according to *Beverage Digest*, an independent company that tracks the global beverage industry. The U.S. bottled water business in 2006 totaled roughly $15 billion, it said.

No timetable was available for when customers will see the label change on store shelves, another Pepsi spokeswoman, Michelle Naughton, told CNN.

Pepsi released a statement saying: "If this helps clarify the fact that the water originates from public sources, then it's a reasonable thing to do."

Coca-Cola does not have plans to change the labeling on its Dasani brand bottled water, a company spokesman told CNN, despite the fact the water also comes from a public water supply.

Dasani's U.S. sales totaled approximately $1.89 billion in 2006, according to *Beverage Digest* calculations.

THE EFFECTS OF DISTILLED WATER

- **Dr. Michael Colgan, Optimum Sports Nutrition**: "Distilled water is the only form of water, which is free from all contaminants and impurities. Distilled water is the only clean water. Virtually everything is removed from the water by steam distillation. Seven brands we tested run from two to twelve PPM contaminants. That's about as clean as you can get."

- **Dr. Clifford Dennison, physical and biological scientist**: "There's no absolute proof that drinking distilled water will remove kidney stones and gallstones, reduce cataracts, or cure emphysema. But there are hundreds of case histories of people who have enjoyed success in alleviating or overcoming these health problems when they began drinking distilled water exclusively."

- **California Department of Consumer Affairs:** "Highly mineralized water has been associated with the formation of (kidney) stones in the urinary system."

- **Dr. Charles Mayo, Mayo Clinic:** "'Water Hardness' is the underlying cause of many, if not all, of the diseases resulting from poisons in the intestinal tract. These (hard minerals) pass from the intestinal walls and get into the lymphatic system, which delivers all of its products to the blood, which in turn, distributes to all parts of the body. This is the cause of much human disease. 'Water Hardness' is inorganic minerals in solution (in water). When these minerals enter the intestines in drinking water, there is an immediate reaction between them and the fats, oils and fatty acids present, causing precipitation of inorganic calcium, magnesium, iron and so on—to form new, insoluble compounds."

- **U.S. Department of Health:** "All kidney machines operate on distilled water."

- **Mark A. Sircus, OMD, director of the International Medical Veritas Association:** "We cannot allow our public water officials to pull a rug over our eyes. We cannot afford to fall back on crude beliefs and basic assumptions but have to examine all sides of the issue and look into the facts. It's a fact that William K. Reilly, administrator of the EPA under the first Bush administration, classified drinking water contamination among the top four public health risks posed by environmental problems. Successful detoxification and chelation are totally dependent on an adequate intake of good water. Water is our body's only means of flushing out toxins. The more water we drink, and the purer and more alkaline that water is, the more we allow our body to purify itself."

- **Dr. F. Batmanghelidj, MD:** "I have treated, with only distilled water, well over three thousand persons with dyspeptic pain. They all responded to an increase in their water intake, and their clinical problems associated with the pain disappeared."

- **Dr. Edward M. Wagner:** "Chronic Fatigue Syndrome sufferers are instructed to drink distilled water."

- **Harvey and Marilyn Diamond,** *Fit for Life II: Living Health*: "Distilled water has an inherent quality. Acting almost like a magnet, it picks up rejected, discarded, and unusable minerals and, assisted by the blood and the lymph, carries them to the lungs and kidneys for elimination from the body. The statement that distilled water leaches minerals from the body has no basis in fact. It doesn't leach out minerals that have become part of the cell structure. It can't and won't. It collects only minerals that have already been rejected or excreted by the cells … To suggest that distilled water takes up minerals from foods so that the body derives no benefit from them is absurd."

- **Dr. Allen E. Banik:** "The only minerals that the body can utilize are the organic minerals. All other types of minerals are foreign substances to the body and must be eliminated. Distilled water is the only water that can be taken into the body without any damage to the tissues. What we as scientists and the public have never realized is that minerals collected in the body from water are all inorganic minerals, which cannot be assimilated (digested) by the body. The only minerals that the body can utilize are the organic minerals (from fruits and vegetables). All other types of minerals are foreign substances to the body and must be disposed of or eliminated. Today, many progressive doctors prescribe distilled water to their patients."

- **Dr. Paul Bragg, N.D. PhD, author of** *The Shocking Truth about Water*: "When distilled water enters the body, it leaves no residue of any kind. It is free of salts and sodium. It is the most perfect water for the healthy functioning of the kidneys (83 percent water). It is the perfect liquid for the blood (83 percent water), the ideal liquid for the efficient functioning of the lungs (86 percent water), stomach, liver (85 percent water), and other vital organs. Why? Because it is free of all inorganic minerals. It is so pure that all liquid drug prescriptions are formulated with distilled water. The greatest damage done by inorganic minerals—plus waxy cholesterol and salt—is to the small arteries and other blood vessels of the brain (75 percent water). Hardening of the arteries and calcification of blood vessels starts on the day you start taking inorganic chemicals (and minerals from tap water) into our bodies."

- **Dr. James Balch, MD:** "There is only one water that is clean. Steam distilled water. No other substance on our planet does so much to keep us healthy and get us well as water does."

- **U.S. Army Health Services Command, Raymond H. Bishop, Jr. MD**: "Distilled water is safe to drink and should have no adverse effects on your health. Distillation merely removes most of the dissolved materials, which are found in all natural waters."

- **United States Department of Agriculture:** "There is nothing about distilled water that would make it harmful for the body. It may be helpful to remember that distilled water is the only water available for crews of naval vessels at sea. The only proven method of correcting cooking and drinking waste pollution in the home is through the use of a home distiller."

- **Dr. Brown Landone, neurologist:** "Hard water seals each cell with a film, so oxygen cannot reach the imprisoned cells. Nature then develops new cells, which thrive on less oxygen. These cells are called cancer cells. Distilled water often frees the imprisoned cells and allows the oxygen to reach these cells."

- **Dr. Joseph Price, famous U.S. medical researcher and author of *Coronaries/Cholesterol/Chlorine*:** "Chlorine is the greatest crippler and killer of modern times."

- **Dr. August Rollier, famous Swiss physician:** "Distilled water, good nutrition, sunshine, fresh air, deep breathing, massage, and exercise. No hard water should ever be given to a patient."

- **Dr. Robert Willix Jr.:** "The best method for purifying your water is a system that distills your water and then carbon filters it"

- **Academy of Natural Healing:** "The contamination is beyond help. More than 55,000 of the regulated chemical dumps across the nation are leaking into the ground water. *Science News*, 1993. With all this in mind, you need to know that distilled water is an excellent source of water. Distilled water is water that has been heated to the boiling point so that impurities are separated from the water, becoming vapor or steam. It is then condensed back into pure liquid form. The impurities remain in the residue, which is simply thrown away. Distilled water contains no solids, minerals, or trace elements, and has no taste. Distillation removes the debris, bacteria, and other contaminants."

- **Center for Disease Control:** "35 percent of the reported gastrointestinal illnesses among tap water drinkers were water related and preventable."

- **Michael McCarthy, water expert:** "Ask yourself what the world's most precious commodity is, and you might say gold; you might say diamonds. You'd be wrong on both counts. The answer is water. If by 'most precious' we mean what's most desired by most people, nothing comes close to water—fresh, clean water, that is."

- **United States Environmental Protection Agency:** "Each year in the U.S., lead in drinking water contributes to 480,000 cases of learning disorders in children and 560,000 cases of hypertension in adult males. 45 million Americans drank water from water systems that fell short of SDWA standards in 1994 and 95."

- **Natural Resources Defense Council:** "Unhealthy drinking water affects children in different ways than it does adults. There is cause for special concern for the health of children who do."

- **Dr. Ron Kennedy:** "As to carbon filtered and reverse osmosis (RO) water, these are better solutions than tap water or mineral water, however they still fall far short of the standard set by distilled water."

- **Ian "Doc" Shillington, ND:** "Don't take unnecessary risks, drink healthy, drink distilled. To be sure, several drinks of local tap water will not kill you, but common sense will tell you that your body cannot function and survive with daily ingestion of poison."

- **Canadian Nutrition Guide:** "The viruses of major concern in relation to drinking water are those of intestinal origin, excreted by infected animals or humans, which reach water resources by way of the soils unlimited potential for serious disease and contamination of the human body."

- **Dr. Alexis Carrel, winner of Nobel Prize in medicine, scientist at the Rockefeller Institute:** "The cell is immortal, renew the fluid at regular intervals and give the cells what they require for nutrition. Premature death and many symptoms of the aging process are due to an accumulation of toxins in the cells of our body."

- **Dr. Andrew Weil, founder of the University of Arizona's Program in Integrative Medicine, which he started in 1994:** "The question as to whether distilled water leaches minerals out of the body reflects another persistent myth. While pure water helps to remove minerals from the body that cells have eliminated or not used, it does not 'leach' out minerals that have become part of your body's cell structure. Neither does distilled water cause your teeth to deteriorate, a false claim made by a filter manufacturer looking to boost sales. As far as acidity goes, distilled water is close to a neutral pH and has no effect on the body's acid/base balance"

- ***American Medical Journal:*** "The body's need for minerals is largely met through foods, not drinking water."

- **Dr. Henry A. Schroeder, Dartmouth Medical School:** "The minerals which the human body needs that are in the water are insignificant to those in food … and anyone simply eating a varied diet, not even a balanced diet, could hardly suffer a mineral deficiency."

FINAL WORD

To make a statement that there is "no, real scientific evidence" concerning water is absurd. Chemists, biologists, and nutritionists around the world agree that inorganic materials create a thin film along both the small and large intestine. The film is like stacking bricks that are attracted to each other. The film attracts another film. It begins to build, forming what is an epidemic to millions of people—constipation—resulting in serious digestive problems. Virus and bacteria grow which create bigger problems—a slowed metabolism, arthritis, gout, hardening of the arteries, varicose veins, as well as others. The thin layer of film thickens and hardens, forming deposits where blood flows the slowest. Scientists around the world have found that the type of water we drink is, in many instances, the culprit.

My sixty-nine-year-old mother drank tap and spring water her entire life. She has had chronic kidney infections throughout her adult years. In her latest bout, she went to speak to her doctor of ten years to get the standard treatment: prescription pills and cranberry juice. While in person, she explained to him that her son (me), now a nutritionist, recommends distilled water as a necessity to pushing out bacteria in a kidney infection. Her doctor replied, "Shirley, distilled water is the only water I would ever drink or recommend, and I should have mentioned it before."

In the 1990s, I watched my own personal workouts get better after drinking one gallon of water. I noticed that I couldn't get the pump if I didn't drink the adequate amount of water mentioned above. I looked very flat and felt tired. My skin doesn't have the tightness to it if I don't drink one gallon of water per day—regardless of whatever critics tell me.

I also found that if I had eaten high amounts of sodium, I would retain more water. I pushed everything out by drinking distilled water. I decided from that point on that water intake is essential in how I feel and look. It's something no doctor can convince me otherwise. The truth is the more water you drink, the more water you lose. The more water and salt you lose, the more your body hardens and the tighter your skin gets. It's something I personally cannot deny.

For the first two weeks, people complain about constantly running to the bathroom—some feel it's unnecessary. I will tell you this. You need to listen to your body. What is happening is your body is detoxing itself. Water, along with other inorganic material, is being flushed out of the body for the first time, particularly with distilled water. This will slow down and subside, but you must not be discouraged. If anything, you should be happy. It's your body's way of removing waste after years of punishment. It gets rid of water it was holding on your ankles, hips, thighs, and belly. You are excreting much more than you realize, not just from your bladder. After two weeks, your body will start to believe water intake is now consistent and will start letting go of areas that it has held on to since you have been in a state of dehydration.

Distilled water can be found at every grocery store in the United States in the bottled water section. It can also be delivered in five-gallon jugs to your home or business. It's my hope in the very near future you will see sixteen-ounce and 1.5 liter distilled drinking bottled water on every shelf in America.

Let me leave you with this final thought. In her book, *The Fat Flush Plan*, Dr. Anne Louis Gittleman says, "Many individuals carry an extra ten to fifteen pounds of water trapped in their tissues. The water contributes to abdominal bloating, cellulite, face, and eye puffiness. It is what my esteemed colleague Elson Haas, MD, calls 'false fat.' That is, the weight is not the result of additional adipose tissue, or true fat, but of excess water." Dr. Gittleman's first solution? Drink more water!

Chapter 7

The Workout

I don't care if you're sixteen or sixty-seven—this chapter will apply to you. Don't skip it. If you are person who can barely get off the couch because you can only think about eating, sit back and listen, you're going to want to comprehend this chapter. Let each word motivate you. I don't want to be a cheerleader, just the messenger. I want you to know that whoever you are, no matter what you look like, it can all change. Skinny or fat, this chapter will apply to you.

How many of you have actually bought a diet or exercise book and taken the time to do the exercises shown? For most of you, it's information overload, filled with unnecessary explanations and hard-to-follow examples. This chapter is different; you will see how simple it is to read. I'm taking a different approach and understand that we need to get right to the point. Every personal trainer in the world wants you to understand this concept. You pay top dollar to have them share it with you.

Eating right will shape your body—working out will sculpt it.

Here is a true story of how eating correctly shaped the body and working out sculpted it. In November 1987, I had a buddy who was out of the country for a few years serving a church mission. He started a diet I put together for him from the other side of the world.

He had taken pictures of himself prior to the day he started my program and sent them to me. After seeing his pictures, I told him I would need ninety days to get him to the leanness he was striving for. He was thirty pounds overweight, with serious love handles, and severe belly fat from eating Mexican food literally every meal for eighteen months. He explained to me that he was addicted to food, but sick of himself. He felt I was the one guy who might be able to help, but he still had his doubts. He wrote back, after I told him how long it would take to see results and said, "It would never happen," and he didn't think he could change his body in ninety days.

Without having weights or a treadmill where he lived, he simply ate cleanly as I instructed him miles from home through letters. On the eightieth day of following the diet, he described how, after living on a dirt floor in South America with no electricity or running water, "he had never looked better, and that his body had changed dramatically." When he arrived home, he wanted to train with weights for another ninety days before leaving for college and asked me to write him up another program.

He was lean and had hardened his body through foods, but still had areas that bothered him. His biggest complaint was his chest. He said he wanted to close the gap in his sternum plate with more muscle, as the pectoral muscles were genetically apart. I explained to him how we would do that through weight training and continuing the diet. Once again, he told me, "Closing the gap between my chests will be an impossibility."

About sixty days later, he called me. He said he could not believe that by doing close grip bench press from all three angles, (flat bench, incline bench, and decline bench) stimulating muscle growth, and keeping him in a positive nitrogen balance through food—he had closed the lifelong gap in his breast plate with muscle. He was astonished. It goes to show how the power of lifting weights with a strategy can actually change the way you look—even when you were given something different at birth.

WHICH PERSON DO YOU WANT TO BE TODAY?

Suppose for a minute you are the person who goes to work and feels overwhelmed with your job. You have no energy or enthusiasm about working out. You really could care less about joining a gym or working out from home. For many people, those feelings are normal. It's human nature. What if though, by eating right as I have outlined, you start to feel a change just weeks into this? What if you actually start wanting to move your body?

I'm going to take you through a series of people; you decide which person you want to be on any given day. There are different levels of fitness to choose from. Person One is someone who has never worked out, or wants to start slowly and just move their body anyway they can. Person Five, is the person who is completely dedicated to working and will do what it takes. It will allow you good and bad days. Remember though, moving at all is good—especially when you eat the way I have instructed in Chapter 8.

Person 1:

1. The goal:

– Walk for twelve minutes, at least three days per week.

2. The facts:

- Realistically, doing twelve minutes of cardio, three days per week would be a good start.

- Moving twelve minutes is twelve times better than doing nothing at all.

- If you do nothing else today, make sure you move for twelve minutes.

- Walking for twelve minutes will start burning calories and glucose—allowing for more glycogen to be stored in the muscle.

- Consistency is the key. Do not take the all-or-nothing approach. You will see results, but they might be slower than you would like.

3. What you can expect:

- Results will depend greatly on your diet and if you are drinking the recommended water intake using primarily distilled water.

4. What you need to understand:

- You will shape your body by doing this workout; however, you must train with weights to sculpt your physique.
- You need to learn two life-changing concepts: interval training and after-burn.

5. Suggested workout plan:

- Walk for twelve minutes on a treadmill or on your favorite trail.
- Walking your dog or a bike ride would be fine.
- Move any way you can for twelve minutes—and don't make excuses.

Person 2:

1. The goal:

- Push-ups.
- Sit-ups (crunches).
- Walk for twenty minutes as hard as you can walk.

2. The facts:

- The human body depletes glycogen between eighteen and twenty minutes on the average.
- For women, the push-up is fantastic. It doesn't create size; it tones and hardens while creating definition.
- Building muscle is not easy; toning up is.

3. What you can expect:

- You can expect to see changes in muscularity and overall body composition.
- You will see results in twenty days, especially eating cleanly each meal.

4. What you need to understand:

 – By enabling your body to exceed a twenty-minute workout and push closer to thirty minutes, you intensify the body fat process.

 – Push-ups are one of the all-time great exercises for the body.

 – By doing just a few push-ups and adding one each time, every workout will create a real sense of wellbeing, as well as building some strength and definition.

 – You can swim, bike, or choose any piece of equipment as long as you move hard for twenty minutes.

5. The suggested workout plan:

 – Start with five push-ups. If you can only do a single push-up, start there.

 – Add one push-up to your last total each time you do this workout.

 – Do one set of thirty crunches—if you don't know what an exercise is, Google it.

 – Immediately after push-ups and crunches, walk for twenty minutes as hard as you can.

 – Walk up a grade to bring your heart rate up quickly—as this is the desired goal.

 – If you are spent after the twelve minutes of going hard on the piece of cardio equipment, call it a day and don't lose sleep over it, tomorrow is a new day.

Person 3:

1. The goal:

 – Introduce interval training to your workout.

 – Work out to failure to create the after-burn.

2. The facts:

 – The June 2008 issue of *Men's Health* states you can achieve more progress in a mere twelve to fifteen minutes of interval training (done three times a week) than that guy grinding away on the treadmill for an hour. "Researchers recently found that intervals burn three times as much fat as running twice as long at a moderately hard, steady pace."

– Interval training is basically walking for two minutes and running for one minute.

– After-burn or EPOC is created when you work each body part to failure as to continue burning calories after your workout is over.

3. What you can expect:

– Quicker results than level two with a better overall tone and composition to the body within two weeks of starting the program.

4. What you need to understand:

– You are trying to dip into (finally) type II muscle fiber, which is fast twitch by moving harder and faster, directly affecting the after-burn. After-burn is burning calories and fat for up to two days after your workout. This is why a sprinter is typically lean and muscular

– This level-three workout plan will change your "set point." The set point is the weight that our body will tend to make us gravitate toward.

– Realize "to failure" means to do each set to where you cannot lift the bar or your own weight any longer.

5. The suggested workout plan:

– Begin the program doing three sets of push-ups to failure.

– After push-ups, do three sets of crunches at sixty reps each.

– Rest for thirty seconds in between sets—regardless of exercise.

– Immediately after the crunches, walk two minutes, then sprint for one minute on a treadmill. If you cannot sprint, walk or jog as hard as you can.

– If you don't like the treadmill, go run in a setting where you feel comfortable.

- You can also choose a stationary bike and add resistance, peddling from slow to fast—do this for twelve minutes straight without stopping.

Person 4:

1. The goals:
- Weight training four days per week, doing one body part per day (one day covers two body parts) to help create the after-burn.
- Twelve minutes of interval training.

2. The fact:
- To maximize after-burn, exercising one body part per week to failure will give you the most energy with the most rest possible for the best results.
- Women should stay with very light weight to create the feminine, lean model-type body.

3. What you can expect:
- If you had a choice between the marathon long distance body or sprinter body, which would it be? You can expect the sprinter body from this program.

4. What you need to understand:
- Doing cardio after weight training pushes all carbon dioxide out to create new cell growth.
- Doing one body part per day—four days a week—will sculpt the body.
- This person works chest one day only, arms the next, legs the next, and back with shoulders the next.
- Four days a week is the key to see real change.
- The reps are as many as you can to failure after choosing a weight that you will not exceed fifty times.
- You will be performing only one set per exercise to failure.

5. The suggested workout plan:

- Mondays: Chest—Incline and decline press. Finish with dips. Each exercise to failure.
- Tuesdays: Arms—Bicep curls and tricep extensions. Each exercise to failure.
- Wednesdays: Off
- Thursdays: Legs—Squats followed with lunges. Each exercise to failure.
- Fridays: Shoulders and back—Military press followed by pull-ups. Each exercise to failure.
- Immediately after weight training, perform a minimum of twelve minutes of interval training. If you cannot interval train (two minutes walk, one minute run), walk as fast as you can for a minimum of twelve minutes with an occasional burst of running.
- When weight training to failure, choose a weight and do not exceed fifty reps per set.

Person 5:

1. The Goal:

- Weight train four days per week using both heavy and light weight for males to shock the body.
- Twelve to twenty minutes of interval training.

2. The Facts:

- Science tells us by weight training with our legs, we release more growth hormone than previously thought.
- Growth hormone creates a leaner, harder physique while burning fat.
- Choosing one body part per day allows the body to break down and repair muscle properly—maximizing body fat loss.
- It's this training with cardio as prescribed that allows for the fastest transformation possible.

3. What you can expect:

- By sculpting the entire body, from the calves to the shoulders, you will look symmetrical.
- The results will be fantastic in a short amount of time doing this workout.
- Serious results are in thirty days. Six weeks could be an amazing transformation, depending on your diet.

4. What you need to understand:

- Heavy lifting is for males who want to achieve a fuller, more athletic look.
- If the female works with heavy weights, she will grow, but not much since the amount of testosterone in her body is much less compared to men.
- You will now (mostly men) incorporate both light and heavy workout days. Doing between four and six reps will add size.
- A release of your body's own growth hormone with the increased leg work is the greatest fat burner of all time.
- Women should stick with light weight. Perform a minimum of three sets; however, five sets per exercise is better.
- The weight-training segment should last about thirty to forty-five minutes.
- The cardio part should be twelve to twenty minutes, but doesn't need to exceed this time. One hour is the maximum you need to exercise.
- This person realizes it's now all about after-burn and not about calories burned during a specific workout.

5. The suggested workout plan:

- **Mondays:** Chest—Incline and decline press and finish with dips. Three sets of each exercise to failure. Men should choose both light and heavy weight.
- **Tuesdays:** Arms—Bicep curls and tricep extensions. Three sets of each exercise to failure. Men should choose both light and heavy weight.
- **Wednesdays:** Off

- **Thursdays:** Legs—Squats followed with lunges to failure, standing toe raises for calves if you have access to it. Three sets of each exercise to failure. Men should choose both light and heavy weight.

- **Fridays:** Shoulders and back—Military press followed by pull-ups. Three sets of each exercise to failure. Men should choose both light and heavy weight.

- **The cardio:** Push yourself twelve–twenty minutes as hard as you can go. You should be sweating when this is over.

What is the exercise after-burn or EPOC?

EPOC (Excess Post-Exercise Oxygen Consumption) or after-burn represents the oxygen consumption above resting level that the body is utilizing to return itself to its pre-exercise state. Rarely have we seen scientific evidence like this validating the particular workout's post-exercise capability to incinerate fat faster.

David Zinczenko may have said it best: "When early studies compared cardiovascular exercise to weight training, researchers learned that those who engaged in aerobic activities burned more calories during exercise than those who tossed around iron. You'd assume, then, that aerobic exercise was the way to go. But that's not the end of the story. It turns out that while lifters didn't burn as many calories during their workouts as the folks who ran or biked, they burned far more calories over the course of the next several hours.

"This phenomenon is known as the after-burn—the additional calories your body burns off in the hours and days after a workout. When researchers looked at the metabolic increases after exercise, they found that the increased metabolic effect of aerobics lasted only thirty to sixty minutes. The effects of weight training lasted as long as forty-eight hours. That's forty-eight hours that the body was burning additional fat."

Zinczenko closes with a powerful bit of information, "The message: aerobic exercise essentially burns only at the time of workout. Strength training burns calories long after you leave the gym, while you sleep, and maybe all the way until your next workout."

- **Chantal A. Vella, PhD & Len Kravitz, PhD, exercise physiology experts:** "Intensity in an aerobic exercise bout has the greatest impact on EPOC. As exercise intensity increases, the magnitude and duration of EPOC increases. Therefore, the higher the intensity, the greater the EPOC and the greater the caloric expenditure after exercise."

- **Jeff Bayer, fitness specialist:** "If your goal is to achieve a maximum fat loss, you will want to optimize EPOC as best as you can, thereby increasing the total number of calories you burn that day. The degree of EPOC you experience has a direct correlation to the intensity of your workout session. The harder you are able to work out, the more you will disrupt all the measures listed above and, therefore, the more energy your body will need to expend to bring them back down to normal once again. Furthermore, there are certain variables within your workout that you can alter to get that after-burn up even higher: When trying to maximize EPOC, taking slightly shorter rest periods will help. This forces your body to work harder without as much recovery between sets, so you will require more in-depth recovery after the session has been completed."

- **Therese Iknoian, an award-winning and internationally published fitness and sports journalist:** "Your body is still burning calories, silently, efficiently, slyly. Even after most exercise if over, calories continue to get gobbled. You probably call it 'after-burn.' For the record, exercise scientists call it 'excess post-exercise oxygen consumption,' EPOC or after-burn. Pretty cool that you can do nothing and still keep the fires burning. But the level, type and length of the something you do before you stop have a big effect on the after-burn."

- **Department of Biological Sciences, Ohio University:** "EPOC or after-burn lasted for up to the duration of forty-eight hours after workout. Proving that EPOC will burn calories up to two days after working high intensity circuit training."

- **Jeff M. Reynolds, PhD:** "Current research of resistance weight training and EPOC has noted a relationship between exercise intensity and elevated metabolic rate. As weight lifting intensity increases, the EPOC duration also increases."

- **Joni Kettunen, PhD:** "With EPOC and training effect, even the beginner can train successfully."

- **Ron Jones, fitness expert:** "The shorter duration and higher intensity intervals work much better to stimulate metabolism, fitness, and promote more rapid fat loss. The idea is that very hard work requires more energy for recovery. Energy=Calories. Therefore, you burn more calories 'after' the workout is done than other more traditional workout designs—this is also called the 'after-burn' effect."

- **Don Hagan, PhD:** "EPOC is related to the intensity and duration of the exercise work bout, i.e., the greater the intensity and the longer the duration of a training session, the greater the EPOC. Thus, a high intensity exercise session will have high EPOC, while low intensity exercise will have low EPOC."

- **Chris Scott, PhD, exercise physiologist at the University of Southern Maine Human Performance Laboratory:** "When exercise ends, it takes time and energy for muscle cells to return to resting levels. Recovery can also be expensive: Depleted glucose and fat stores need to be refilled, accumulated cell products need to be removed and protein levels need to be built back up. All this requires energy. And the more rebuilding to be done, the greater the rate of EPOC, which in turn means more calories (using fatty tissue as fuel) are being burned after your workout. While the primary factor in determining EPOC is exercise intensity, so is duration—just not to the same extent. Intense exercise is associated with a tremendous amount of fat breakdown. The higher the exercise intensity, the greater the amount of carbohydrate burned. But the energy requirements of recovery, especially an active recovery, need to be considered. To be sure, muscle uses mostly carbs during weight training, but all the fat that's broken down during exercise is subsequently used to fuel recovery. EPOC primarily depends on fat and lactic acid as fuel. In fact, the recovery from EPOC is almost all aerobic and a terrific oxidizer of fat."

FINAL WORD

ABC's Diane Sawyer hired celebrity trainer Jim Karas for her personal training goals. Karas said, "You can kiss your treadmill goodbye." He says cardiovascular workouts burn a few calories, but far fewer than you think. From 1987–2000, the number of people exercising on treadmills increased by 900 percent; meanwhile obesity doubled. "If your true goal is to lose weight, interval strength training is the only way to go."

Whether he knows it or not, Karas is teaching about afterburn or EPOC. Although I don't agree with him about getting rid of your treadmill, he obviously understands the benefit of strength training and how it affects the human body days after exercise. He stresses that weight training to failure is the key regardless of the weight chosen. He is spot-on with most of what he says, however, know that if you are trying to really pack on weight, the heavier you use, the bigger you get. It's the law of physics. So pick a weight that will suitable to what your goal is.

If you want to be lean with very little size, chose a weight that is very light with a minimum of twenty-five reps to failure. If your goal is to gain size, do reps between four and six times as heavy as you can go while not exceeding or going beneath. Either way, you will be strength training and allowing the effects of the after-burn to take place. The harder you push yourself, the greater the EPOC. For the ultimate lean physique, strength train to failure with at least twelve minutes of high intensity aerobics such as using a treadmill with or following the weight training with minimal rest between sets. It will create havoc on body fat and create the body you have always wanted, I can personally attest to that.

WHAT EACH WORKOUT LEVEL DOES FOR THE BODY:

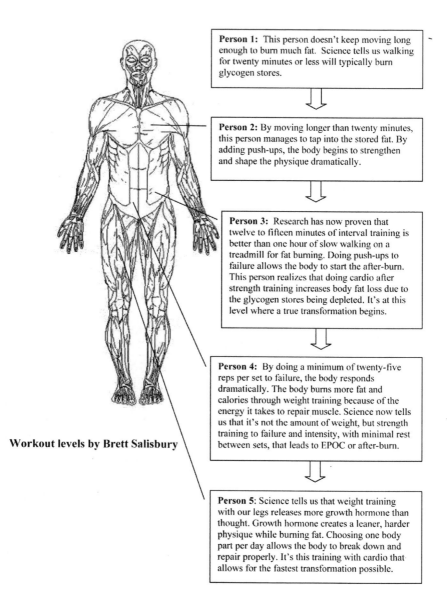

Person 1: This person doesn't keep moving long enough to burn much fat. Science tells us walking for twenty minutes or less will typically burn glycogen stores.

Person 2: By moving longer than twenty minutes, this person manages to tap into the stored fat. By adding push-ups, the body begins to strengthen and shape the physique dramatically.

Person 3: Research has now proven that twelve to fifteen minutes of interval training is better than one hour of slow walking on a treadmill for fat burning. Doing push-ups to failure allows the body to start the after-burn. This person realizes that doing cardio after strength training increases body fat loss due to the glycogen stores being depleted. It's at this level where a true transformation begins.

Person 4: By doing a minimum of twenty-five reps per set to failure, the body responds dramatically. The body burns more fat and calories through weight training because of the energy it takes to repair muscle. Science now tells us that it's not the amount of weight, but strength training to failure and intensity, with minimal rest between sets, that leads to EPOC or after-burn.

Person 5: Science tells us that weight training with our legs releases more growth hormone than thought. Growth hormone creates a leaner, harder physique while burning fat. Choosing one body part per day allows the body to break down and repair properly. It's this training with cardio that allows for the fastest transformation possible.

Workout levels by Brett Salisbury

Chapter 8

What It Will Take to Transform

On Tuesday, November 27, 2007, Colorado State University's Denise Palmeri said, "Ketosis is a dangerous result of high protein diets. It can lead to gout, kidney stones, or the nasty breath odor about which some protein dieters complain. Not all protein diets are low enough to induce ketosis under fifty grams of carbs."

WHAT IS HER BEST ADVICE?

"Choose a diet that allows at least fifty grams of carbs to prevent ketosis."

Does that advice sound familiar?

The amount of carbohydrates, proteins, and fats—to a very large degree—affects how you look. How well you can balance and measure these three will determine the appearance of your physique. It really is as simple as that. You can change your body, your metabolism, and even put muscle where there was none before. You are now empowered with knowledge from the previous seven chapters and it's time to put it in action all the scientific evidence and get right to the point.

If you are opening the book and starting with this chapter because you want to see how to transform, I would ask that you wouldn't. You need to prepare yourself mentally with the knowledge I have supplied by reading the previous chapters leading up to this moment, so that you may understand why I'm writing so specifically for each meal since they are based on scientific evidence using thousands of subjects.

From this point on, it's time to change the way you think. *Eat to live—do not live to eat.* It's going to take the first four weeks from your starting date to change your metabolism along with learning some valuable tricks to help your metabolism burn at a high rate, day or night. If you are the person who has been eating horribly for the past twenty years, it will take four weeks to do some damage on those fat deposits. This plan will do just that.

THE MEAL PLAN

Treat these meals like a prescription. Take them every three hours. Don't miss times. If you do miss, don't double up. If you take the prescription as prescribed, you will get the results you were expecting.

For most of you, meals one and two are all going in a blender. It's so easy and quick, it takes two minutes and you're out the door. It's a reality for the working class. If you have time to prepare a meal, even better, more power to you. I just don't believe it's feasible for most Americans.

As for the whey protein discussed in chapter 5, without question *Muscle Milk* by Cytosport is superior on all accounts. Especially their chocolate flavor. Women, don't be turned off by the title "muscle milk". It's not going to bulk you up, it will however, lean you out. As for the taste? Once you try this product, all others fail miserably by comparison. This is the one protein powder that even women cannot deny. In fact when you buy the container, smell the inside of it. You will quickly understand why it's going to be different. It's also going to save your diet, you will feel like you're cheating with this stuff. What's amazing is that 2 scoops (a male serving) is equivalent in carbohydrates to a half of a banana. Yet a banana won't fill you up and has more sugar. However, with this protein and added fiber you will feel full for the next three hours and begin the transformation of your life.

Why I like this particular protein is that Cytosport uses protein blends which is used for both daytime and evening meals unlike many other protein powders on the market. It blends both whey and casein proteins. Whey protein is digested and absorbed quickly which fills your blood with amino acids rapidly, inhibiting muscle breakdown. Casein proteins have a slower rate of absorption and digestion. Casein basically supplies amino acids over a longer period of time to your brain and muscle. Both should be used in conjunction throughout the day. What makes this stuff special is that the makers patterned it after human mother's milk which has essential antioxidants, vitamins and minerals called Colostrum. Bovine Colostrum, is high in antibodies and is produced in female mammals during the first 24 to 48 hours after birth. Bovine colostrums is identical to that found in human colostrums but at higher levels. Colostrum also contains high concentrations of leukocytes, protective white cells which can destroy disease-causing bacteria and viruses. The powder is high in Potassium and is significant in Vitamin C as well as many other vitamins and minerals. It's also lactose free, which many others are not.

One fat used in the powder is medium-chain triglycerides or MCT's. These are the predigested, "fast-burning fats," which are more likely burned for muscle energy and heat that stored as fat. The protein also uses long-chain polyunsaturated fatty acids, which are also less likely to be stored as fat. Of total lipids, human mother's milk contains approximately 20% MCT's. Muscle Milk replicates this important lipid structure.

After putting the ingredients into a blender, you will need a grinder. A grinder is necessary to grind your flaxseed. You can buy flaxseed at any health food store. I also like flaxmeal which is already pre-ground and tastes great. My personal favorite is Bob's Red Mill brand. Next is old fashion oats. I get Quaker, but other brands are fine. Do *not* buy instant packets. The food makeup is different, and the insulin will spike when it enters your bloodstream. You need the kind you would cook on a stove for five minutes. You will also need a measuring cup. Don't think you can guess—it will kill the diet. Mix it all with water—more or less, depending on the consistency you want. Do the math.

Between the canister of protein, the oats, and flaxseed, this will be cheaper than fast food. It ends up being between two and three dollars per meal.

Here is something very important ...

When you blend this, the more ice, water and flaxseed you add, the less sweet it tastes. You can also buy shakers from a health food store. They actually have a little metal ball inside the plastic part and you can literally put all your ingredients in this dry. Get in your car and go. You simply need to add water and mix with your hand. No electricity needed. One powder that seems to be going over very well is Gold Standard Whey Cookies and Cream. Again a small reminder. I will be coming out with a powder that contains the big 3 for both men and women, and it will taste fantastic. I have decided that blending and grinding are not convenient forcing me to take action and to create a powder that will make all of this simple as I put all ingredients in one packet. www.TransformDiet.com will keep you updated on this.

<u>MEAL 1</u>: FOR THE MALE

- ½ cup raw oats.
- One tablespoon of ground flaxseed.
- 2 scoops of whey protein.
- Sixteen ounces of distilled water to drink.
- Blend everything into a blender with water using ice. I wouldn't recommend using milk for the first twelve weeks of this program (see Chapter 1).
- If you insist on using fruit at this point, you can add either five blueberries or three strawberries. No bananas as they have too much sugar. Also, remember that flaxseed and protein have a few carbs as well.

OR

- ½ cup of oatmeal slow cooked on the stove, not microwaved at it affects insulin in the body.

- Sprinkle one tablespoon of ground flaxseed over oatmeal. You can sweeten the oatmeal with one packet of artificial sweetener if you wish. Do not use table sugar as it will store fat—artificial sweeteners do not.

- Two whole eggs with five egg whites cooked on the stove however you like them.

- Sixteen ounces of distilled water to drink.

OR

- Low carbohydrate, low to little gluten bread found at health food stores (Ruisleipa bread from Finland is the best). The total amount of bread slices cannot exceed thirty grams. Do not use a typical store-bought brand. Ezekiel bread is not recommended. When in doubt, stay away from these breads (Chapter 1).

- Fresh salmon (about eight ounces, but no more).

- Treat this meal like lox and bagels. Place salmon on top of the bread and enjoy.

OR

- If you need variety or have a special diet, eat a protein, carbohydrate, and fat, staying within the prescribed amount. I do not recommend deviating with your own choices for the first twelve weeks; it usually leads to failure of seeing drastic results if you give yourself too many choices. Keep it simple.

Male total: Forty-six grams of carbohydrates, forty grams of protein, eighteen grams of monounsaturated/polyunsaturated fat. (Depending on what protein powder you buy changes these numbers)

Why meal 1 is so good for the male

The raw oat will enter the blood stream as a low-glycemic index food (Chapter 5).

The flaxseed will help slow entry of carbohydrates, forcing the stomach to separate carbohydrates from protein and fats (Chapter 5).

There will be minimal insulin excretion from the pancreas as these two foods keep spikes from occurring (Chapter 3).

The BV-rated 104 protein of whey will be absorbed faster than the egg, which will move glycogen quickly into the muscle, but will not get a spike from insulin due to fiber from oats and flaxseed (Chapter 4).

The flaxseed will also balance testosterone, moving it in favor of estrogen and will not allow a conversion to take place, due to the extremely powerful lignan hormone (Chapter 5).

If the estrogen-to-testosterone levels are swaying one way or the other, the phytoestrogen lignan helps in balancing this out. This is what creates muscle hardness and definition, and rids stubborn belly fat as testosterone wins the "seesaw" battle (Chapter 5).

The carbohydrates stay below fifty grams, allowing the metabolism to burn up at its maximum capacity, not allowing the metabolism to overwork and slow down (Chapter 3).

The protein intake is sufficient and will start the body into a positive nitrogen balance, that is, to start building muscle, and not allowing muscle to be used as a source of fuel (Chapter 4).

The sixteen ounces of distilled water help to push everything through the cell—ridding inorganic material doesn't allow one organ like the liver help the kidney in its function (Chapter 6).

The mix of these three foods eaten everyday for four weeks will drop leptin levels dramatically, allowing for the first cheat meal after the four weeks are complete (Chapter 3).

<u>MEAL 1:</u> FOR THE FEMALE

- ½ cup of raw oats.
- One tablespoon of flaxseed.
- 1 scoop of whey protein.
- Sixteen ounces of distilled water to drink.
- Blend into a blender with water using ice. I wouldn't recommend using milk for the first twelve weeks of this program. Powders

taste as good as smoothies now and water will give it a great consistency (Chapter 5).

OR

- ½ cup of oatmeal slow cooked on the stove, not microwaved since it affects insulin in the body (Chapter 3).
- Sprinkle one tablespoon of ground flaxseed over oatmeal. You can sweeten the oatmeal with a packet of artificial sweetener since it has no effects on insulin or body fat.
- Two whole eggs with two egg whites cooked on the stove.
- Sixteen ounces of distilled water to drink.

OR

- Low carbohydrate, low to little gluten bread found at health food stores (Ruisleipa bread from Finland is the best). The total amount of bread slices cannot exceed thirty grams. Do not use a typical store-bought brand. Ezekiel bread is not recommended. When in doubt, stay away from these breads (Chapter 1).
- Fresh salmon (about four ounces, but no more, half the size of your fist).
- Treat this meal like lox and bagels. Place salmon on top of the bread and enjoy. Make sure that the bread does not exceed sixteen grams per slice.

OR

- If you need variety or have a special diet, eat a protein, carbohydrate, and fat, staying within the prescribed amount. I do not recommend deviating with your own choices; it usually leads to failure from seeing drastic results.

Female total: Thirty-eight grams of carbohydrates, twenty-two grams of protein, twelve grams of monounsaturated/polyunsaturated fat. (Depending on what protein powder you buy changes these numbers)

Why meal 1 is so good for the female

The oat—whether cooked or raw—may have even more benefits to a woman (Chapter 5).

With higher levels of estrogen, she has higher levels of body fat (Chapter 5).

Oats not only speed the metabolism—they work on cellulite. The flax balances estrogen levels and pushes out any excess (Chapter 5).

Too much estrogen floating in the body can cause breast cancer; flaxseed can change that (Chapter 5).

Women seem to store more fat on the hips and thighs than men do—fiber and good fats change that (Chapter 5).

The "big three" (flax, oat, and whey) combined may work faster because of the estrogen-to-testosterone ratio in women. The lignans control this and now help burn fatty tissue (Chapter 5).

You simply see results because of the new hormonal balance being brought to the body (Chapter 5).

The sixteen ounces of distilled water help to push everything through the cell—removing inorganic material and allowing the kidneys and liver to do their intended jobs (Chapter 6).

The mix of these three foods eaten every day for four weeks will drop leptin levels dramatically, allowing for the first cheat meal after the four weeks are finished (Chapter 3).

MEAL 2: FOR THE MALE

- ½ cup raw oats.
- One tablespoon of flaxseed.
- 2 scoops of whey protein.
- Blend in a blender with water using ice.
- Sixteen ounces of distilled water to drink.

OR

- Eat a protein, carbohydrate, and fat, staying within the prescribed formulas.

    Male total: Forty-six grams of carbohydrates, forty grams of protein, eighteen grams of monounsaturated/polyunsaturated fat

Why meal 2 is so good for the male

Eating three hours after the first meal is key to keeping your metabolism on fire (Chapter 2).

By eating flaxseed three hours later, you really start to allow the lignans to play a serious role on hormonal balance for both men and women (Chapter 5).

The body will change these hours if you allow it (Chapter 2).

You will not be hungry until lunch since the fiber and fat tell your brain you are full. If you can consistently eat this meal, you will see incredible results (Chapter 5).

MEAL 2: FOR THE FEMALE

- 1/4 cup of raw oats.
- One tablespoon of flaxseed.
- 1 scoop of whey protein.
- Blend all ingredients in a blender with water and ice.
- Sixteen ounces of distilled water to drink.

OR

- Eat a protein, carbohydrate, and fat of your choice (staying within the prescribed formulas).

    Female total: Twenty-four grams of carbohydrates, twenty grams of protein, eleven grams of monounsaturated/polyunsaturated fat

Why meal 2 is so good for the female

The oats—whether cooked or raw—may have even more benefits for women (Chapter 5).

With higher levels of estrogen, she has higher levels of body fat. Oats not only speed the metabolism, they work on cellulite (Chapter 5).

Whey protein has so many benefits for women—there are too many positives to list here (Chapter 5).

MEAL 3: FOR THE MALE (LUNCH)

- Order two sushi rolls, but ask the chef to change the middle part of a rainbow roll to tuna. They typically fill it with artificial crab or something else.

- Ask for spicy tuna. Spice gives it more flavor and the sauce in the middle will not affect body composition.

- Order one roll with rice and the other roll without rice.

- If you order two rolls of sushi and do not remove the rice from one of the rolls, you are now close to ninety grams of carbohydrates in one meal, which will spike insulin and slow the metabolism, as fifty grams is about the maximum the body can handle in a three-hour period.

- This will be the perfect balance of protein, carbs, and fats. (This meal can be eaten three days per week)

OR

- At a Thai restaurant, order any curry dish with chicken. Add the curry sauce to taste and keep on the side as the sauce should be used in moderation with rice. Iced tea is allowed, but do not use table sugar. No sodas are allowed for twelve weeks. You can eat this meal twice per week.

OR

- At American restaurant chains, order a salad with dressing on the side (oil and vinegar is best).
- Order a meat of your choice such as steak, chicken, or fish. I like grilled salmon with rice or potato for lunch.
- Be sure the potato is about the size of a small red potato, which is the total amount of carbs you are allowed.
- I would order red meat only twice per week for cholesterol and saturated fat reasons. Drink with water or iced tea.

OR

- Stir fry with one teaspoon of olive oil, with favorite meat.
- The amount of rice cannot exceed fifty grams, which is about one cup of cooked rice or half a cup uncooked.
- Do *not* eat uncooked rice.

OR

- Two ounces of spaghetti noodles with six hard-boiled eggs. After the noodles and eggs have been cooked, add a teaspoon of olive oil and salt and pepper to taste with either lettuce, or spinach leaves. You can also add mixed vegetables like broccoli with the pasta while it boils. It's delicious.
- It can be eaten every day at lunchtime, but not after (until you get where you want). Instead of weighing the noodles every

time, you can simply grab a handful of noodles. If one end of the bunch is the size of a nickel, it is roughly two ounces.

- Although pasta noodles are a high-glycemic index food, when mixed with olive oil, the rate that carbohydrates are metabolized is slower, keeping the insulin from spiking. It's the oldest trick in the book. You can easily hard-boil the eggs the night before along with the pasta. Simply add olive oil, salt and pepper, and reheat it at work. You can also choose any meat to mix with noodles. Red meat should only be eaten twice per week.

OR

- Drink a protein shake with the big three as prescribed earlier.

OR

- Eat a protein, carbohydrate, and fat, staying within the prescribed formulas.

Male totals: fifty grams of carbohydrates, forty grams of protein, and seven grams of monounsaturated/polyunsaturated fat

Why meal 3 is so good for the male

Let me focus on the sushi for now—the rice is a high-glycemic index food and would have normally entered the bloodstream by itself too quickly. However, by eating it with salmon, it will slow insulin response and not allow a spike to occur (Chapter 5).

Remember, fat slows the rate at which carbohydrates enter the bloodstream—making salmon an excellent choice since it's high in the fatty acid Omega-3. Fat does not affect insulin either way (Chapter 5).

The Omega-3 found in salmon is a different Omega-3 than flaxseed. It is a tremendous fat burner and will wreak havoc on fatty tissue (Chapter 5).

The Japanese eat rice in every meal. They are one of the leanest cultures in the world. They eat a high-glycemic index food every meal (rice), but they are lean because they usually incorporate a meat with the dish and cook with oil. Protein slows the absorption rate of carbohydrates, like fat does. Don't let American folklore convince you that white rice under fifty grams per meal is a bad thing—it's not. To put this in perspective, one banana has thirty-nine grams of carbs. Rice is an excellent choice since it expands in the stomach, prevents overeating, is gluten free, and contains no fructose (Chapter 5).

MEAL 3: FOR THE FEMALE (LUNCH)

- One sushi roll: Here is what you will order from the chef. Ask the chef to change the middle part of a rainbow roll to tuna. They typically fill it with artificial crab or something else. Ask for spicy tuna.

- Spice adds more flavor and the sauce in the middle will not affect body composition.

- Order one roll. This is about forty-five grams of carbohydrates— this is a little more than you should have, however it will be your last starch carb meal of the day (at least for the first twelve weeks).

- This will be the perfect balance of protein, carbs, and fats.

- Order this three days per week.

OR

- At Thai restaurants, split the meal in half. It's the perfect size for women and can be used for another meal.

- Order any curry dish with chicken. Add the curry sauce to taste and keep on the side.

- Use the sauce in moderation with rice.

- Drink water or iced tea.

- No sodas are allowed for twelve weeks.

OR

- At American restaurant chains, cut the meat portion in half and save it for another day.
- Order a salad with dressing on the side.
- Order a meat of your choice such as steak, chicken, or fish.
- Grilled salmon with rice or potato is a good choice for lunch.
- Be sure the potato is about the half the size of one small red potato—this is the total amount of carbs you are allowed.
- I would order red meat only twice per week for cholesterol and saturated fat reasons.
- You would be able to order a salad with oil and vinegar, but keep it basic.
- Drink with water or iced tea. Do not sweeten iced tea with real sugar. Artificial sugars do not effect external body composition.

OR

- Rice with your favorite meat.
- Stir fry with one teaspoon of olive oil.
- The amount of rice cannot exceed thirty-five grams for women, which is about three-quarters of a cup of cooked rice or a quarter-cup uncooked—salt and pepper to taste.
- Do *not* eat uncooked rice.

OR

- A little less than two ounces of spaghetti with four hard-boiled eggs—two without yolks. Eat two yolks per day. After cooking the noodles and eggs, add a teaspoon of olive oil and salt and pepper to taste with either lettuce or spinach leaves. You can also add mixed vegetables like broccoli with the pasta while it boils. It's delicious.
- It can be eaten every day at lunchtime, but not after (until you get where you want). Instead of weighing the noodles every time, you can simply grab a handful of noodles, look at one end of the bunch and it should be no larger than the size of a penny—this is roughly 1 ½ ounces.

OR

- A protein shake with the big three as prescribed earlier.

OR

- Eat a protein, carbohydrate, and fat, staying within the prescribed formulas. If you need variety or have a special diet, you will have good results by not exceeding the recommended allowance.

Female totals: fifty grams of carbohydrates, twenty grams of protein, and six grams of monounsaturated/polyunsaturated fat

Why meal 3 is so good for the female

Let me focus on the sushi for now, the rice is a high-glycemic index food and would have normally entered the bloodstream by itself too quickly. However, by eating it with salmon, it will slow insulin response and not allow a spike to occur (Chapter 5).

Remember, fat slows the rate at which carbohydrates enter the bloodstream, which is also found in salmon, but do not affect insulin either way (Chapter 5).

The fish is high in Omega-3s. This is a different Omega-3 than flaxseed. It is a tremendous fat burner and will wreak havoc on fatty tissue (Chapter 5).

The proteins in fish in this state are excellent for the body (Chapter 4).

The Japanese eat rice in every meal. They are one of the leanest cultures in the world. They eat a high-glycemic index food every meal (rice), but they are lean because they usually incorporate a meat with the dish and cook with oil. Protein slows the absorption rate of carbohydrates, like fat does. Don't let American folklore convince you that white rice under thirty-five grams per meal is a bad thing—it's not. To put this in perspective, one banana has thirty-nine grams of carbs. Rice is an excellent choice since it expands in the stomach, prevents overeating, is gluten free, and contains no fructose (Chapter 5).

MEAL 4: FOR THE MALE

- This is where the switch is made to completely eliminate starch carbohydrates, except those found naturally in the whey protein powder which is the key to this entire way of living, at least until you see the results you want. By doing this, your body cannot pull glucose from your muscle—it is forced to work on body fat all afternoon and evening long. That is why as the evening progresses you are in fat-burning mode right up to until bedtime.

- You can have fibrous carbs (spinach, broccoli, or leafy greens).

- *Minimal starch.* That being said, it becomes really easy to grab another shake with two scoops of protein, this time without oats.

- Since this meal is around 3:00 PM, or three hours after lunch, it will be your final shake of the day. Add almonds to this to replace the flaxseed. Do not exceed twelve almonds for this meal.

- Mix all contents in water. Let me make this clear. If a shake is not want you want, then don't have one. You need to find a protein with monounsaturated fat here with minimal starch.

- Maybe a salad with chicken again, but I can't stomach three salads per day. It doesn't work for me. Remember—convenience and nutrition are the key here—along with great taste.

- You can eat all the fibrous carbohydrates you wish.

- Beware of tomatoes—as they are technically a fruit. They have higher levels of sugar and should be used in moderation for at least the first twelve weeks. If you insist on tomatoes, have one small or five cherry per day up until lunch.

- I would steer clear completely of corn and carrots. Remember that it's not always about the internal effects on the body, but the combination of both. They do a body good internally, but create belly fat externally on many of us. Use in moderation.

Male totals: Eighteen grams of carbohydrates, thirty-eight grams of protein, sixteen grams of monounsaturated/polyunsaturated fat

Why meal 4 is so good for the male

By not eating starch carbohydrates after lunch, your body will begin the dip into fat (Chapter 4).

The depleted levels of carbohydrates are where the body fat reduction will begin (Chapter 3).

Protein also plays a role in decreased hunger (Chapter 4 and Chapter 5).

MEAL 4: FOR THE FEMALE

- This is where the switch is made to completely eliminate starch carbohydrates, except those found naturally in the whey protein powder which is the key to this entire way of living, at least until you see the results you want. By doing this, your body cannot pull glucose from your muscle—it is forced to work on body fat all afternoon and evening long. That is why, as the evening progresses, you are in fat-burning mode right up until bedtime (Chapter 3).

- You can have fibrous carbohydrates (spinach, broccoli, or leafy greens).

- *Minimal starch.* That being said, it becomes really easy to grab another shake with one scoop of protein, this time without oats.

- As this meal is around 3:00 PM, or three hours after lunch, it will be your final shake of the day. Add almonds to this to replace the flaxseed. Do not exceed twelve almonds for this meal.

- Mix all contents in water. Let me make this clear. If a shake is not want you want, then don't have one. You need to find a protein with monounsaturated fat with minimal starch.

- Maybe a salad with chicken again, but I can't stomach three salads per day. It doesn't work for me. Remember, convenience and nutrition are the keys here—along with great taste.

- You can eat all the fibrous carbohydrates you wish.

- Beware of tomatoes—as they are technically a fruit. They have higher levels of sugar and should be used in moderation at least for the first twelve weeks. If you are insistent on tomatoes, have one small or five cherry per day before lunch.

- I would steer clear completely of corn and carrots. Remember that it's not always about the internal effects on the body, but the combination of both. They do a body good internally, but create belly fat externally on many of us. Use in moderation.

Female totals: Eleven grams of carbohydrates, twenty grams of protein, ten grams of monounsaturated/polyunsaturated fat

Why meal 4 is so good for the female

By not eating starch carbohydrates after lunch, your body will begin to dip into fat (Chapter 4).

The depleted levels of carbohydrates are where the body fat reduction will begin (Chapter 3).

Protein also plays a role in decreased hunger (Chapter 4 and Chapter 5).

<u>Meal 5:</u> For the male

- Do not worry about salt intake, but don't overdo it; you will flush it out with the amount of distilled water you're drinking.
- You may also use hot sauces or herbs. Be careful with salsa. You can use mustard in moderation.
- No ketchup, mayonnaise, or butter with any meal.
- You cannot eat deli turkey or chicken.
- Minimal starch carbohydrates are allowed, until you get where you want. However, you can still obtain great results by eating starch of less than twenty grams if needed, but I would wait for the first twelve weeks.
- I recommend two cups of a fibrous carbohydrate. I use a sauce called Soyaki—a teaspoon of the product will enhance every meal. Find products like this that really give flavor to your meal. Don't overdo and be a very careful about any types of spreads. They can prevent you from getting where you want. Read the labels for carbs—they sneak up on you.

- Take all the ideas from the previous four meals and remove any starch carb and replace with a fibrous carb.
- I like a salad or stir-fry with chicken, fish, or the occasional steak. I also like hardboiled eggs with fibrous carbs.
- Occasionally, have a lunch meal for dinner—it can help in times when you are struggling.
- If you are going to cheat, don't do it at this time—earlier in the day is a better choice. If you do cheat, don't lose sleep over it, regroup and make your next meal count—just remember how leptin works (Chapter 3).

Male totals: Eight grams of carbohydrates, forty grams of protein, six grams of monounsaturated/polyunsaturated fat.

Why meal 5 is so good for the male

- By not eating starch carbohydrates after lunch, your body will begin the dip into fat-burning mode while you sleep (Chapter 4).

MEAL 5: FOR THE FEMALE

- Do not worry about salt intake, but don't overdo it; you will flush it out with the amount of distilled water you're drinking.
- You may also use hot sauces or herbs. Be careful with salsa. You can use mustard in moderation.
- No ketchup, mayonnaise, or butter with any meal.
- You cannot eat deli turkey or chicken.
- Minimal starch carbohydrates are allowed, until you get where you want. However, you can still obtain great results by eating starch of less than twenty grams if needed, but I would wait for the first twelve weeks.
- I recommend two cups of a fibrous carbohydrate. I use a sauce called Soyaki—a teaspoon of the product will enhance every meal. Find products like this that really give flavor to your meal. Don't overdo and be a very careful about any types of

spreads. They can prevent you from getting where you want. Read the labels for carbs—they sneak up on you.

- Take all the ideas from the previous four meals and remove any starch carb and replace with a fibrous carb.

- I like a salad or stir-fry with chicken, fish, or the occasional steak. I also like hardboiled eggs with fibrous carbs.

- Occasionally, have a lunch meal for dinner—it can help in times when you are struggling.

- If you are going to cheat, don't do it at this time—earlier in the day is a better choice. If you do cheat, don't lose sleep over it, regroup and make your next meal count—just remember how leptin works (Chapter 3).

Female totals: Eight grams of carbohydrates, twenty grams of protein, six grams of monounsaturated/polyunsaturated fat.

Why meal 5 is so good for the female

- By not eating starch carbohydrates after lunch, your body will begin the dip into fat-burning mode while you sleep (Chapter 4).

<u>MEAL 6:</u>

– This meal is not recommended unless you are the lean body type looking to add muscle. This meal can also be for the male or female who might be especially hungry one night. I recommend this meal to someone over three hundred pounds in the beginning, as it will help you to not struggle with hunger pains.

- One scoop of protein for the male. For the male trying to build muscle, take two scoops—or one scoop if you are simply satisfying a hunger pain.

- One scoop of protein for the female.

- Do not add flaxseed if you have already had four tablespoons. Do not exceed this amount per day.

- Take five almonds with your protein shake.

- Do not eat starch or fibrous carbohydrates.

- Women get four ounces of meat and men get eight ounces.

- After twelve weeks, non-fat cottage cheese could be an occasional good choice here due to its carb-protein-fat ratio. Also, the fact that it's a casein protein can help you sleep better. However, do not exceed a half-cup at anytime.

- Find a protein choice with no carbs that works for you.

FINAL WORD

1. You will get headaches in the beginning. Remember your body is detoxing between the foods you are eating and the water intake. You are cleansing yourself and getting rid of waste. The body responds with headaches. Eating junk food before you started this diet is probably the culprit. This usually lasts three to five days then ends.

2. Decreased hunger. By eating fiber (from flaxseed, whey, and oats), proteins, and fats, your body will not be hungry by combining all three. You will be amazed by this. It will be the first program you have ever been on that feels like this. It's the trick of fiber and good fats, along with eating every three hours. Increasing the amount of carbohydrates in your first three meals is essential. For example, simply adding another quarter-cup of oats at breakfast can end any hunger pains by dinner. Try it and see if I'm correct.

3. Increased urination and bowel movements. Again, it's the body's way of removing toxins and waste. These will continue as long as you eat cleanly, but will subside to a regular cycle after about twenty days.

4. You will experience a sense of wellbeing. Seven days after starting, you will feel on top of the world. It's the one item on this list I can't prove. It's the one you will soon have days after living this program.

5. You are not snacking on things like peanuts—which is an absolute joke in so many other diets. You will not be hungry.

6. You will have lower bad cholesterol, higher good cholesterol, regular blood pressure, and triglycerides below 150 after sixty days. You will also have excellent blood chemistry with lower body fat and more stamina, higher energy, and a better immune system. Do a before and after with your doctor with all these tests. You will see the drastic changes in twelve weeks.

7. Buy a very good multivitamin, but never take it on an empty stomach. It can have trouble metabolizing and can upset your stomach.

8. If you try not to deviate much from the recommended foods I give and eat them day in and day out for twelve weeks—you will transform. That being said, once you reach your desired body fat and weight, you can add starch carbohydrates after lunch. I would never exceed fifty grams of carbohydrates per meal. By doing so, you will look and feel fantastic for life. Most importantly don't let the fat grams in double digits concern you. Simply stay below 18 grams of the right fats and it will all come together.

9. When drinking the recommended distilled water set by the Institute of Medicine and the Mayo Clinic—the goal is one gallon for males and ninety-one ounces for females—you simply drink water at room temperature since this makes it easier to drink throughout the day. By drinking 1 gallon of distilled water each day as this pushes unwanted sodium out of the body to really allow the body to tighten up not allowing for "false fat" to accumulate.

10. Be sure to eat within thirty minutes of waking up. This will start your metabolism since it's been in starvation mode and shut down while you slept.

11. Here is a great trick for a tough day or days. Remember, you don't want to think about this as a diet, it needs to be a way of life. When your third meal (lunch) is starting you need to go eat as clean as you can, but eat until you really are full. Don't get down on yourself for this either. Don't skip meals 4 and 5 because of the over eating at meal 3. This is the biggest mistake you can make and will again force the body into starvation mode. On meals 4 and 5 you now get back to cutting down the starch carbs. You will also not feel deprived as you can dip into foods at lunch time that you are craving, allowing yourself to be strong every evening which is the key to hardening the body. Don't eat starch carbs after 2:00pm unless they are found naturally in your protein shake and you will see results.

12. And now, let's put this all together—what will it take to transform?

WHAT IT WILL TAKE TO TRANSFORM

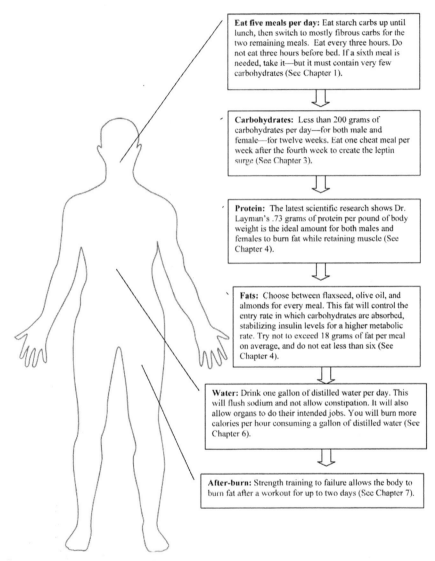

Eat five meals per day: Eat starch carbs up until lunch, then switch to mostly fibrous carbs for the two remaining meals. Eat every three hours. Do not eat three hours before bed. If a sixth meal is needed, take it—but it must contain very few carbohydrates (See Chapter 1).

Carbohydrates: Less than 200 grams of carbohydrates per day—for both male and female—for twelve weeks. Eat one cheat meal per week after the fourth week to create the leptin surge (See Chapter 3).

Protein: The latest scientific research shows Dr. Layman's .73 grams of protein per pound of body weight is the ideal amount for both males and females to burn fat while retaining muscle (See Chapter 4).

Fats: Choose between flaxseed, olive oil, and almonds for every meal. This fat will control the entry rate in which carbohydrates are absorbed, stabilizing insulin levels for a higher metabolic rate. Try not to exceed 18 grams of fat per meal on average, and do not eat less than six (See Chapter 4).

Water: Drink one gallon of distilled water per day. This will flush sodium and not allow constipation. It will also allow organs to do their intended jobs. You will burn more calories per hour consuming a gallon of distilled water (See Chapter 6).

After-burn: Strength training to failure allows the body to burn fat after a workout for up to two days (See Chapter 7).

The Transform Diet by Brett Salisbury

Chapter 9

———⟫◆⟪———

My Favorite Tricks

A true transformation for the man or woman takes place when you involve more than just diet and exercise. These tricks allow for a true head-to-toe transformation. Here are those tricks. The list is in no particular order. I have no agenda and no ties to any of these companies.

1. The Antiperspirant-Deodorant trick: I have had a few friends over the years that, regardless of what deodorant or antiperspirant they use, it didn't seem to help. I eventually would let them in on the secret. It's a good one. It actually came from my cousin (Rob Lennon). So, here it is and here is how you need to do it. This may sound a little fanatical, but for many people, it's needed.

Immediately after showering and cleaning yourself, you step out and towel dry off. Before doing anything else, reach for the Mitchum antiperspirant roll-on. Do not use the white chalky choice, since it will leave residue on your armpit—a nasty look we often see. Deodorants do not work. They simply hide the odor in the beginning and then blend together with whatever smell or funk you might have. Have you ever smelled somebody who had a combination of smells? For instance, a Ralph Lauren perfume mixed with body odor. How is that? Unscented Mitchum changes all of that and prevents the perfume or cologne wearer from mixing smells.

Do not get anything *but* unscented. No matter what anyone tells you, lying next to your spouse or significant other with the smell of their underarm deodorant—not to mention body odor—can unknowingly cause irritation and headaches.

2. The body hair trick: This one is a good one. Do you really like seeing women—or men for that matter—with a ton of arm or body hair? This trick I learned from a teammate of mine (Mike Salido) while playing football at BYU. The clippers you get for your haircut? They have different attachments. Take the shortest attachment and begin cutting your arms, legs, pubic area, and armpit, whatever. Here is the beauty of it. You will never cut the hair to its root. It will still be there—only shorter. In fact, it will be so short that, even with dark hair, it becomes natural looking. No shaving, no mess, no stub.

By using this trick, the body looks cleaner and the skin looks tighter; it also shows more definition. Also, remember those little dingle balls in your armpit caused by the white chalk from the deodorant? Simply cut the armpit down to the shortest attachment, leaving armpit hair, yet it's so tight you can hardly see it.

Don't let your spouse or significant other tell you how great body hair is. It's okay in moderation. But, when you resemble Grizzly Adams? Not good. I also don't like the look of completely shaved legs on anyone but a female. This is the answer.

3. Tres Flores/Three Flower trick: This $4 bottle of hair product will last two to six months, depending on how much you need. You apply it after you get out of the shower. If you are a guy with dry hair or a woman with split ends, this stuff does the trick. Do you want your hair to stay in place and not move much—but still not be oily, greasy, or stuck like hairspray? Beautiful. The stuff is made by Pfizer in New Jersey. It has two applications. One is a liquid oil form, not the one I recommend. However, I recently found out the Hispanic community loves it. The oil application has a stronger flower smell than the wax. Stick to the wax. The great thing is that when it rains or when you sweat, it doesn't run into your eyes and burn. Sebastian, Nexus, and so many others try to make this product and don't come close. They also charge you $30 per bottle.

4. Mouthwash, toothpaste trick: There is not a person on the planet that likes bad breath. Here is a trick that may sound like it is not a big deal, but it is. You will never have fresher breath in a short amount of time. Immediately when you get out of bed and before your shower, fill up the Listerine or the comparable store brand and fill the black cap halfway. Put it in your mouth. Instead of focusing everywhere around the mouth, leave it on your tongue. If you think your tongue isn't the real issue—think again. It's where all the bacteria and bad breath congregate. Please don't let the critics tell you that alcohol will dry your mouth out. You can explain to them that nearly one gallon of distilled water per day hydrates the driest mouths on a daily basis.

Anyway, let the Listerine begin burning your tongue. That's crucial. Immediately grab your toothbrush, while leaving the mouthwash in your mouth, and brush your teeth. After thirty to forty-five seconds, spit out the mouthwash. After that, immediately grab your tongue scraper. If you don't know what a tongue scraper is—Houston, we have a problem. Next, spit out the mouthwash and scrape your tongue at least five times. Next, grab your toothbrush and do what you normally due with toothpaste, and brush your teeth as you normally would. I would recommend flossing too, but that may be for later that night. Trust me when I tell you your breath has never smelled or been fresher in two minutes.

5. Hexahydrate trick: I love this trick. Tired of "pitting"? (It's when your armpits sweat and leave the sweat rings in the under arm of the shirt). It affects men and women every day. It's broken up relationships. It's also destroyed many shirts. Want to be done permanently with armpit sweat? Here is the trick. First, know that as good as Mitchum is, it cannot prevent this problem. Don't let any commercial tell you their antiperspirant can either. Hexahydrate is prescription only. Let me tell you though, if you don't know how to apply it, you will think it doesn't work either.

Here's the catch. At night—hopefully after a shower—lie down. By lying down, your glands actually shut off underneath your armpit. Did you catch that? If you stand and apply this stuff, it will not work and you will sweat. I know it sounds crazy but you have to be horizontal. Anyway, as you're laying down getting ready for bed, you apply underneath both armpits. It's powerful. You may even burn a little in the first minute, but that will go away soon. Next, go to sleep. Do not remove. It needs to work for about five hours.

No surgeries needed and no more embarrassing rings at the office. I have really seen this one change lives. This stuff will last up to three weeks in one application before you need to re-apply it. For some, this may be the best trick yet.

6. Selsun Blue trick: Ever heard of sunspots? They are not a real big deal, but can be a burden. It's actually a fungus that affects millions every day. You need to buy Extra Strength Selsun Blue. Apply for ten minutes every day for two weeks. The white spots will go away. You know if you have them by tanning—the area will look like it has white blotches. It works and it's powerful. Knowing this will save you from the doctor prescribing the same thing.

MY FINAL WORD

It's now proven that our thoughts are so powerful they can make our physical bodies ill and unable to perform properly. A recent study has shown that human beings have over 60,000 thoughts per day, 80% of them are negative. So be careful how and what you think. Take control of your thoughts.

I memorized this when I was eleven years old. I read it in the local paper while growing up. I don't know if a day has gone by that I have not thought about it. I know from that day forward, I was never the same again. Remember, no matter what anyone says, you can do anything in life including transform:

"Our thoughts are ultimately going to manifest themselves in some way. So, if you're coming from a success conscience, success has to follow, it's as simple as that. The trick is to not let all the doubts, fears,

and opinions submerge you, but to turn your heel, and say, 'Wrong, I'm on my course now—nothing and no one can stop me.'"—Dyan Cannon

Index

A

abdominal fat (visceral fat), 23

abs development, 3, 40

The Abs Diet (Zinczenko), 1, 6–8, 23

Academy of Natural Healing, 69

Aceto, Chris, 15

acidity (pH), 42

aerobic exercise, compared to weight training, 84, 85. *See also* cardio

after-burn, 78, 79–81, 83–88, 111. *See also* EPOC

Agatston, Arthur (*The South Beach Diet*), 1–2, 3, 4, 5, 118

ALA (Alpha-linolenic acid), 48, 49

albumin (protein in blood plasma), 28

allergies

    to food, 40, 42

    to milk, 2

almonds

    in The Abs Diet, 8

    benefits of, 38–39

    as good fat, 38–39

    recommended amount of, 38

    in Transform Diet, 104, 105, 108

Alpha-linolenic acid (ALA), 48, 49

American Academy of Dermatology, 49

American Cancer Society, 54

American Heart Association, 11

American Journal of Clinical Nutrition, 4, 35

American Medical Journal, 71

amino acids, 2, 27, 29, 51, 54

Andersen, James W., 43

antibodies, in bovine colostrum, 91

antibody creation, and whey protein, 55

antioxidants

    in almonds, 38

    in breast milk, 91

    in fruit, 4

    in lignans, 45

antiperspirant-deodorant trick, 113

Antonio, Jose, 46

anxiety, relief of, from flaxseed, 49

apples, 18

Arkansas Children's Nutrition Center, 55

arthritis, 49, 72

arteriosclerosis, 68, 72

artificial sweetener, 93, 102

asparagus, 18

Atkins, Robert (*The Atkins Diet*), 23

The Atkins Diet (Atkins), 1, 15, 23, 29, 31, 33

autoimmune diseases, 37

avocados, 39

B

bacon, 7, 31

bad breath, 30, 115, 118

Badger, Thomas, 55

Balch, James, 69

bananas, 49, 90, 92, 101

Banik, Allen E., 68

Barlow, Jim, 33

Batmanghelidj, F., 67

Bayer, Jeff, 85

BCAA (branched chain amino acid), 33, 54

bench press, 76, 82, 83

Bergin, Michael, xii

beta-carotene, 39, 49

bicep curls, 82, 83

biking, 79

Biological Value (BV) rating system, 52

Bishop, Raymond H. Jr., 69

blenders, 90

blood pressure, 43, 60

blood sugar

effect of excess carbohydrates on, 12, 15

effect of five solid meals on, 5, 9–10

effect of flaxseed on, 49

effect of whey protein on, 53

hypoglycemia, 28

blood vessels, calcification of, 68

blueberries, 92

Bob's Red Mill brand, 91

body chemistry, 29, 30

body composition, 33, 54, 78, 80, 98, 101, 102

body fat

and blood glucose level, 13–14, 29

compared to muscle, 8

effect of carbohydrates on, 11–12, 13, 14, 15, 16

effect of excess estrogen on, 48

effect of fruit on, 5

effect of good fats on, 37, 39

effect of leptin on, 25

effect of lignans on, 47

effect of metabolism on, 30

effect of processed cereal on, 8

effect of protein on, 28, 33, 34

effect of The Abs Diet on, 6

effect of Transform Diet meal plans on, 26, 36, 104, 105, 106, 109, 110

effect of Transform Diet workouts on, 79, 82, 87

effect of waiting until hungry to eat on, 10

effect of whey protein on, 53, 54

effect on metabolism, 22

as endocrine organ, 22–23

and insulin level, 13–14

body hair trick, 114

body hardening

Transform Diet and, 3, 37, 39, 44, 73, 78, 110

and water intake, 72–73

body sculpting, 75, 81, 83

body shaping, 75

body temperature, effect of metabolism on, 31

body tone, effect of Transform Diet workout on, 78, 80

boiled water, 64

Bonds, Barry, 44–45

Boschmann, Michael, 59

bottled water, 65

bovine colostrum, 91

bowel movements, 44, 109. *See also* constipation; Irritable Bowel Syndrome

Bragg, Paul (*The Shocking Truth about Water*), 68

brain function, 30

branched chain amino acid (BCAA), 33, 54

breads, 34, 93, 95

breast cancer, 45, 48, 54, 96

breast milk, 41, 51, 55, 91

Brigham Young University, 114, xi

British Nutrition Foundation, 29

broccoli, 18, 45, 99, 102

brown rice, 18

buckwheat, 45

burn therapy, and whey protein, 55

butter, 106, 107

Buzzle.com, 51

BV (Biological Value) rating system, 52

Byron, Katy, 65

C

calcification of blood vessels, 68

calcium, 35–36, 49

California Department of Consumer Affairs, 66

caloric intake, 8, 10, 15, 26, 34

calorie-counting, cautions of, 10

Canadian bacon, 7

Canadian Nutrition Guide, 71

cancer

and flaxseed, 46, 48, 49

and lignans, 45

prevention of colon cancer, 42

and whey protein, 55

crunches, 78, 79, 80
cucumbers, 18
curry dish with chicken, 99, 101
cyanogenic glycosides, 48
Cyrosport, 90
cysteine, 54
cytokines, 46

D

dairy products
  and abs development, 3
  cautions with, 8
  cottage cheese, 109
  described, 2
  as example of proteins, 28
  lactose intolerance, 2
  milk, 94
  milk allergy, 2
  proteins in, 51
Dartmouth Medical School, 71
decline bench press, 76, 82, 83
de-ionized water, 64
deli chicken, 106
deli turkey, 106
Demark-Wahnefried, Wendy, 46
Dennison, Clifford, 66
detoxing, 109
diabetes
  rates of, 4, 14
  and soluble fiber, 42
  and whey protein, 53, 55
Diamond, Harvey (*Fit for Life* and *Fit for Life II*), 2, 68
Diamond, Marilyn (*Fit for Life* and *Fit for Life II*), 2, 68
dietary fiber, 38
dips (in workout), 83
Discover, 12–13
disease, and distilled water, 67
distilled water
  availability of, 73
  described, 60–63, 65
  effect of, 66–71, 72, 73
  in Transform Diet, 78, 92–97 *passim*,

106, 107, 110, 111, 115
drinks
  iced tea, 99, 101
  juices, 3
  sodas, 99, 101
  water. *See* water
Duke University, 46
dyspeptic pain, 67

E

Eades, Michael R., 29
Eat This Not That Diet, 1
eating
  frequency of, 6–7, 15
  timing of, 4–5, 18, 23, 110
  until satisfied, 5
eating clean, 7
ectomorph, 5
edema, 28
eggs
  amino acid profile compared to whey protein, 51
  and BV (biological value) rating system, 52
  in Transform Diet, 93, 95, 99, 102
electrolytes, 58, 62, 63
emphysema, 66
Enter The Zone, 1
Environmental Protection Agency (EPA), 63, 67, 70
EPOC (Excess Post-Exercise Oxygen Consumption), 85, 86, 87, 88. *See also* after-burn
estradiol, 48
estrogen, 38, 46–48, 49
Excess Post-Exercise Oxygen Consumption (EPOC), 85, 86, 87, 88. *See also* after-burn
exercise. *See also specific exercise modes*
  effect of amount of, 20, 86
  factors contributing to metabolic increases, 84
  and glucose, 77, 86
  and glycogen stored in muscle, 19

and high-protein diet, 33–34
and lower-protein diets, 34
and metabolism, 86
and Transform Diet, 58, 75–89
and whey protein, 53–55
exercise intensity, and EPOC, 86
exercising to failure, 80, 81, 87, 88

F

false fat, 73
Farquhar, John W., 14
fast-burning fats, 91
fat cells, characteristics of, 22
The Fat Flush Plan (Gittleman), 73
fat storage, 12, 21. *See also* body fat
fats
    butter, 106, 107
    and carbohydrates, 37
    fast-burning fats, 91
    good fats, 1, 37–40
    intake of, 89
    low-fat diet, 11, 12, 15
    olive oil, 39, 100
    in raw whey, 52–53
    types of, 36–37
fatty acids, 29, 37, 42, 46, 48, 91. *See also* Omega-6 fatty acid; Omega-3 fatty acid
FDA (Food and Drug Administration), 42
females
    recommended carbohydrate intake, 24
    recommended protein intake, 36
    Transform Diet meal plans for, 94–110 *passim*
    workout specifics for, 83
fiber, 39, 41–42, 52
fibrous carbohydrates, 18, 104, 105, 106, 107
filtered water, 64
fish, 28, 93, 95, 99, 102, 103
Fit for Life (H. Diamond and M. Diamond), 2

Fit for Life II: Living Health (H. Diamond and M. Diamond), 68
flat bench press, 76
flaxseed
    benefits of, 44–45, 49
    breakdown of, 50
    as compared to psyllium, 45–46
    effect on women of, 47–48
    ground flaxseed compared to flax oil, 48
    and lignans, 45
    preparation of, 91
    with raw oat and whey protein, 52
    recommended intake of, 38, 48
    side effects of, 48–49
    in Transform Diet, 93, 94, 95, 97
foliate, in avocados, 39
food, as a drug, 10
food allergies, 2, 40, 42
Food and Drug Administration (FDA), 41, 42
Food and Nutrition Board of the National Research Council, 32
food costs, 92
food measurement, 10, 91
food pyramid, 13, 35
foods. *See specific types*
Franz-Volhard Clinical Research Center, 59
frequency, of eating, 6–7, 15
Friedman, Jeffrey M., 25, 26
fructose (fruit sugar), 3, 4, 21
fruits
    apples, 18
    avocados, 39
    bananas, 49, 90, 92, 101
    blueberries, 92
    cautions about, 3–4, 5, 21
    juicing fruit, 3
    nutrient content of, 4
    as starch carbohydrate, 18
    strawberries, 18, 92
    tomatoes, 18, 104, 105–106
    in Transform Diet, 92, 104
    wild compared to grocery store, 4

effect of instant oatmeal on, 91
effect of juicing fruit on, 3
effect of slow-cooked oatmeal on, 44, 93, 95
and fats, 100
and fiber, 52
jobs of, 15
and leucine, 34–35
and metabolism, 3
and protein, 28, 31
and whey protein, 53
insulin resistance, 14
International Medical Veritas Association, 67
International Society of Sports Nutrition, 46
interval training, 79, 80, 81, 82, 86, 87, 88
ion exchange, 52–53
Iowa State University, 19, 20
iron, 39
irritability, and flaxseed, 49
Irritable Bowel Syndrome, 45–46

J

Jhon, Mu Shik (*Significant Liquid Structures*), 60–61
Johnson, Richard, 4
Jones, Marion, 44
Jones, Ron, 86
Joujon-Roche, Greg, 15
Journal of Applied Physiology, 53
The Journal of Clinical Endocrinology and Metabolism, 59
The Journal of Nutrition, 34
Journal of the National Cancer Institute, 48
juicing fruit, 3

K

Karas, Jim, 87
Kennedy, Ron, 70
Kent State University, 32
ketchup, 106

ketogenic diet, 29, 30
ketone bodies, 29
ketones, 30
ketosis
    and The Atkins Diet, 23
    described, 15, 16, 28–29
    Jay Robb on, 30–31
    prevention of, 89
Kettunen, Joni, 86
kidney problems, 29, 66, 67, 89
Kivinen, Tarpila S., 45
Kravitz, Len, 85

L

lactase (enzyme), 2
lactoferrin, 55
lactose (milk sugar), 2, 3, 52–53
Ladd, Gregg, 6, 28
Landone, Brown, 69
Lanou, Amy Joy, 29
Layman, Donald K., 33, 34, 35, 54
leafy greens, 18
Lemon, Peter, 32, 33, 35
Lennon, Rob, 113
leptin (hormone), 20, 24–26, 107
lettuce, 18, 99, 102
leucine (amino acid), 33, 34, 35, 54
leukocytes, 91
Life Science, 33
lignans
    antioxidants and, 45
    benefits of Transform Diet on, 97
    described, 46, 47, 96
    from flaxseed, 38, 45, 46, 47–49
lima beans, 48
lipids, 22, 91
liver glycogen, 19, 21
liver problems, 29
Lopez, Hector, 46
low-carbohydrate diets, 13, 28, 29, 31
low-fat diet, 11, 12, 15
Ludwig, David, 14
lunges, 82, 84
lupus, 49

lutein, 39

M

Maffetone, Phil, 12

magnesium, 38, 49

males
  recommended carbohydrate intake, 23–24
  recommended protein intake, 33, 36
  Transform Diet meal plans for, 36, 90, 92–110 *passim*
  workout specifics for, 82, 83

man breast syndrome, 47

manganese, 49

marathon body, compared to sprinter body, 81

Mathern, Jocelyn, 47

Mayo, Charles, 67

Mayo Clinic, 67

mayonnaise, 106, 107

McCarthy, Michael, 70

McDonald, Lyle, 25

McKevith, Brigid, 29

McMaster University, 32

MCTs (medium-chain triglycerides), 91

meal plans
  for the female on Transform Diet, 94–96, 97–98, 101–103, 105–106, 107–109
  food costs, 92
  frequency of eating, 36, 90
  for the male on Transform Diet, 92–94, 96–97, 98–100, 104–105, 106–107, 108–109
  and Transform Diet, 111
  your own choices of, 93, 95

measurement
  food, 10, 91
  waist, 10–11

meats, 7, 27, 28, 31, 34, 99, 100, 102

Medical News Today, 22

Medina, Jed, xii

Mediterranean countries, diet of, 37

The Mediterranean Diet, 1

medium-chain triglycerides (MCTs), 91

Men's Health, 6, 79

metabolism
  and body temperature, 31
  and carbohydrates, 23
  effect of body fat on, 22
  effect of complex carbohydrates on, 18
  effect of dairy products on, 2, 8
  effect of exercise on, 86
  effect of fruit on, 5
  effect of high-fiber cereal on, 8
  effect of less than three hours between meals on, 6
  effect of water intake on, 59
  and insulin, 3
  and ketosis, 31
  and lack of muscle, 30
  and leptin, 25, 26
  and protein, 28, 32, 33, 36
  starvation mode, 10
  and Transform Diet, 26, 90, 94, 96, 97, 98, 110

micro-filtration, 52

migraines, 49

military press, 82, 84

milk, 2, 51, 94. *See also* breast milk; lactose (milk sugar)

millet, 45

Mitchum antiperspirant, 113

ModelMax, xii

moderately high-protein diets, 33, 34

Molecular Water Environment Theory (Jhon), 60

monosaturated fats, 36, 37, 39

mouthwash, toothpaste trick, 115

MS (multiple sclerosis), 49

mucilage, 49

multivitamin, 110

muscle fiber, type II, 80

muscle glycogen, 19, 21, 29, 104, 105

Muscle Milk, 90–91

muscle/muscle mass
  compared to body fat, 8
  and frequency of eating, 15

processed cereal, 8
progesterone, 47
prostate cancer, 46
protein intake
    and exercise, 33–34
    high-protein diets, 28, 29, 31
    lower-protein diets, 34
    moderately high-protein diets, 33, 34
    recommended intake, 32, 36
    in Transform Diet, 93–108 *passim*
protein malnutrition, 28
protein powders, 3, 30, 51, 53, 90–91,
    92, 94, 104, 105
protein shakes, 100, 103, 104, 105, 108
protein synthesis/growth, and whey
    protein, 54
proteins
    and absorption of carbohydrates,
        101, 103
    in almonds, 38
    and body fat, 28, 33, 34
    BV (Biological Value) rating system,
        52
    and calcium, 35–36
    casein, 51, 53–54, 55, 91, 109
    controversy about, 27, 32
    in dairy products, 51
    described, 27
    examples of, 27–28
    in flaxseed, 49
    importance of, 28
    and insulin, 28
    and ketosis, 89
    leptin, 25
    and metabolism, 28, 32, 33, 36
    and muscle, 30
    soy proteins, 52
    and Transform Diet, 109, 111
    USDA requirements for, 32
    whey protein, 51–55, 90–91, 92–
        105 *passim*
psoriasis, 49
psyllium, as compared to flaxseed,
    45–46
public water supply (P.W.S.), 66

pull-ups, 82, 84
push-ups, 78, 79, 80, 88

R

rainwater, 61, 63
raw oats. *See* oats, raw
raw water, 63
Reaven, Gerald, 11–12
recovery (from workout), 86–87
red meats, 31, 99, 100, 102
Reichenberg-Ullman, Judyth, 2
Reilly, Keith, 43–44
Reilly, William K., 67
reps, 80, 81, 82, 83, 87
rest periods, 85
reverse osmosis, 61, 64, 70
Reynolds, Jeff M. (researcher), 86
rheumatoid arthritis, 49
rice, 18, 34, 99, 102
Robb, Jay, 15, 30–31
Robertson, Donald S., 59
Rockefeller University, 25, 26
Roizen, Michael (*You: The Owner's
    Manual*), 9
Rollier, August, 69
Roth, Ruth A., 28
Rozen, Michael, 60
Ruislcipa bread, 93, 95
rye, 18, 42, 45

S

salads, 99, 102, 104, 105
Salida, Mike, 114
salmon, 93, 95
salsa, 106, 107
salt intake, 7, 8, 106, 107
saturated fats, 2, 36, 37
sausage, 31
Sawyer, Diane, 87
Schenkenberg, Marcus, xii
Schroeder, Henry A., 71
ScienceDaily, 4, 42, 58, 60, 65
SCN (thiocyanate), 48
Scott, Chris, 86

Printed in the United States
152215LV00006B/20/P